List of contributors

P. Ian Andrews FRACP
Paediatric Neurologist, Sydney Children's Hospital, Randwick and
Senior Lecturer, School of Paediatrics, The University of New South
Wales, Australia

John Beveridge AO, FRACP
Emeritus Professor of Paediatrics, The University of New South Wales,
Australia

Hans H. Bode MD Saarland, FRACP, DABP, DABPE
Paediatric Endocrinologist, Sydney Children's Hospital, Randwick and
Professor of Paediatrics and Head of School of Paediatrics, The
University of New South Wales, Australia

Stephen Cooper FRACP
Paediatric Cardiologist, Children's Hospital Medical Centre,
Australia

Jagdish M. Gupta MD, FRCPE, FRACP, DCh
Visiting Professor of Paediatrics, The University of New South Wales,
Australia

Gad Kainer MB BS, FRACP
Paediatric Nephrologist, Sydney Children's Hospital, Randwick,
Australia

Stephen Koder MB BS, FRANZCP
Staff Specialist Psychiatrist, Prince of Wales Hospital, Australia

John D. Mitchell MB BS Melb., FRACP
Paediatric Gastroenterologist, Sydney Children's Hospital, Randwick
and Senior Lecturer, School of Paediatrics, The University of New
South Wales, Australia

John R. Morton MB BS Adel., FRACP, FARCGP, FCCP
Paediatric Respiratory Physician, Sydney Children's Hospital, Randwick and Conjoint Lecturer, School of Paediatrics, The University of New South Wales, Australia

Anne M. Turner MB BS, FRACP
Clinical Geneticist (H.G.S.A. certified), Sydney Children's Hospital, Randwick, Australia

Marcus R. Vowels AM, MB BS Syd., MD UNSW, FRACP
Director of Department of Haematology and Oncology and Head, Bone Marrow Transplant Programme, Sydney Children's Hospital, Randwick and Conjoint Associate Professor, School of Paediatrics, The University of New South Wales, Australia

John B. Ziegler MB BS Syd., FRACP
Paediatric Immunologist, Sydney Children's Hospital, Randwick and Conjoint Associate Professor, School of Paediatrics, The University of New South Wales, Australia

Preface to the first edition

Multiple choice question examinations have become the accepted norm for assessment of undergraduate and postgraduate students because they are considered to test a wide range of topics, are easier to mark and provide objectivity. The marks awarded do not depend on the whims, moods and fancies of the examiners. Computer analysis of the results allows rapid processing of large numbers of candidates and produces results within a short time of the collection of papers. The statistical analysis of the performance of the paper as a whole as well as the performance of good students compared to those of poor students allows planning of further strategies in teaching. However, the setting of these questions requires a considerable amount of work prior to the examination in order to avoid ambiguity and personal bias of the examiners.

At The University of New South Wales, the School of Paediatrics has used multiple choice questions for more than 15 years. The questions were supplied by the staff of the School and the Prince of Wales Children's Hospital. The questions were scrutinized by an examination committee and their suitability was tested by computer analysis of the results. Over this period we have accumulated more than 1000 questions. The questions in this book were selected from this bank of questions. More questions were added in subject areas which were felt to be deficient.

The critiques were written with the aim of stimulating the student to think rather than simply recall information. Additional information is provided which facilitates further learning and problem-solving abilities.

It is obvious that this book would have been impossible to produce without the tremendous amount of work put in by our colleagues at the School of Paediatrics, The University of New South Wales and Prince of Wales Children's Hospital to whom we are extremely grateful. Unfortunately space does not permit us to thank them individually. We would also like to acknowledge the help of our secretaries, Lillan Holgate and Liz Noakes, for preparing the manuscript and Professor H.H. Bode for writing the foreword.

J.M. GUPTA
J. BEVERIDGE

Preface to the second edition

Since its publication 2 years ago, its popularity has made it necessary to reprint *MCQs in Paediatrics*. In the meantime there have been great advances in paediatrics, especially in the fields of neonatology, genetics, gastroenterology and social medicine. In this edition the chapter on genetics and metabolic disorders has been completely rewritten and new questions have been added in all chapters. Furthermore our colleagues in the various specialities have actively contributed in the preparation and revision of this edition. In order not to increase the size of the book substantially some old questions have been deleted.

Although it was not intended, the book is increasingly being used by students preparing for the MRCP Part 1 and by other higher degree candidates. Many of these examinations include basic sciences. In order to meet the needs of these readers, we have also included in the book some questions on basic sciences which have clinical application.

We would like to acknowledge the help of Ms Carol D'Arcy for keeping up to date the MCQ bank and Mrs Toni Benton for typing the manuscript.

J.M. GUPTA
J. BEVERIDGE

1 Growth and development

1.1. A head circumference measurement falling on the 10th percentile for a given age indicates that

A   ten percent of normal children of the same age would have the same measurement.

B   the patient's head circumference is 10% below the mean value for the age.

C   the patient's head circumference is 10% above the lower limit of the normal range.

D   ten per cent of normal children of the same age would have a head circumference greater than that of the patient in question.

E   ten per cent of normal children of the same age would have the same or smaller head circumference.

1.2. In regard to growth during gestation

A   babies born at 38 weeks' gestation weigh more at birth on average than those born after 42 weeks' gestation.

B   size at birth correlates better with maternal stature than paternal stature.

C   hormonal influences on growth are independent of fetal sex.

D   the peak increase in fetal weight occurs during the third trimester.

E   twins achieve their maximum weight velocity by 32 weeks' gestation.

1.3. Which of the following statements is/are correct?   → they are all

A   Babies are able to respond to sounds *in utero*.

B   Full-term babies are unable to follow a large object at birth with their eyes.

C   A 6-week-old infant would be able to follow a large object through an arc of 135°.   → up to 180°

D   Growth velocity of the head decreases with age.

E   A 12-month-old infant who keeps falling when starting to walk is likely to have cerebral palsy.

1

1.1. E
When quantitative measurements are arranged in order of ascending magnitude, the percentile points refer to values falling on or below that centile.

1.2. A B C D E
After 40 weeks' gestation the placenta develops infarcts and is unable to maintain adequate nutrition of the infant. Epidemiological studies have shown that size at birth correlates better with maternal than paternal stature. There is very little production of testosterone in fetal life and therefore it has no effect on fetal growth. During the last trimester of pregnancy the fetus gains in weight because of deposition of fat. It has been shown that weight velocity decreases after the 'litter' has achieved a certain weight, which is at 32 weeks' gestation for twins.

1.3. A C D
Babies respond to sound *in utero* as demonstrated by changes in heart rate. At birth full-term babies will follow a human face or a large red ball with their eyes. A 6-week-old infant will follow a large object through an arc of 180°. Head growth is maximum in the first year of life and decreases progressively thereafter. Infants tend to keep falling when learning to walk.

1.4. Compared with the body proportions of a 5-year-old child, the newborn infant has

A   a larger head.
B   a larger liver.
C   shorter extremities.
D   a larger mandible.
E   smaller tonsils.

1.5. Which of the following may be normal?

A   A one-week old baby whose weight is the same as at birth.
B   The anterior fontanelle which is larger in size at 2 months than at birth.
C   An 11-month-old infant who has no teeth.
D   An 18-month-old well baby who is not eating.
E   A 4-year-old boy who is frequently touching his penis.

1.6. Compared with older children, full-term infants at 1 month have

A   a higher risk of Gram-negative infections.
B   a smaller risk of iron deficiency anaemia.
C   higher fluid requirements per kilogram of body weight.
D   a smaller surface area per kilogram of body weight.
E   a larger head size compared with body length.

1.7. A normal 4-week-old infant

A   is in danger of suffocation if nursed prone.
B   has a Moro reflex.
C   needs 20 hours of sleep in a day.
D   can distinguish his mother from other people.
E   will follow a large object to the midline.

1.8. A 6-week-old infant

A   will roll over.
B   puts out his arms to be picked up.
C   is able to turn his head towards a loud noise.
D   will regard the human face.
E   holds his head up momentarily in the prone position.

1.4. A B C E

Compared with the body proportions of a 5-year-old child, the newborn infant has a larger head, larger liver and shorter extremities. The mandible has the same proportions, though it is smaller than in a pubescent child. Lymphoid tissue (including tonsils) grows from birth to puberty and then involutes.

1.5. A B C D E

Most infants lose weight after birth and reach their birth weight by the end of the first week. At birth the anterior fontanelle may appear small as a result of over-riding of sutures. Eruption of teeth is very variable and is not by itself an indication of abnormality. In the second year of life the baby eats poorly because of other distractions. It is also the period when growth decelerates and causes anxiety to parents. Masturbation in young children is normal behaviour.

1.6. A B C E

Compared with older children, infants at 1 month have a higher risk of Gram-negative infections because they have no maternal or acquired immunity against these organisms. They are at no risk of iron deficiency anaemia (unless there has been bleeding) because of iron stores derived from the mother and have higher fluid requirements per kilogram of body weight because of their higher metabolic rate. Their surface area per kilogram of body weight is greater and their head is larger compared with their body length.

1.7. B E

Although there is an increased incidence of sudden infant death syndrome in the prone position, a 4-week-old infant is at no risk of suffocation as the infant will be able to lift its head and turn to the side. The Moro reflex is easily elicited. Infants vary widely in the amount of sleep they require. The infant is attracted by the human face (this may be a diagram on cardboard) but does not distinguish between different people. Full term infants can follow large objects with their eyes at birth.

1.8. D E

A 6-week-old infant will follow a human face, but not a small light, through an arc of 180°, will not put out his arms to be picked up until the age of 5 months and is unable to turn his head towards a loud noise, though he may show evidence of hearing. In the prone position the infant can hold his head up momentarily but cannot roll over.

1.9. By the age of 4 months most infants

A   can roll over.
B   have conjugate eye movements.
C   reach out and grab objects.
D   sit with support.
E   have two incisor teeth.

1.10. Which of the following developmental attainments is/are appropriate for a full-term infant at the age of 6 months?

A   Sits but needs to be propped.
B   Reaches with a strong hand preference.
C   Fixes but does not follow a moving face.
D   When placed prone on a table lifts his head and supports the upper trunk on extended arms.
E   Has a brisk, symmetrical Moro response.

1.11. In which of the following conditions are infantile body proportions seen in a 5-year-old child?

A   Malnutrition.
B   Osteogenesis imperfecta.
C   Untreated congenital hypothyroidism.
D   Achondroplasia.
E   Down syndrome.

1.12. A 30-week (7-month)-old infant would be expected to

A   transfer an object from one hand to the other.
B   be toilet trained.
C   clap hands in imitation.
D   be distressed by the approach of strangers.
E   be able to sit up.

1.13. Which of the following skills would be expected of a 7-month-old infant but not a 5-month-old infant?

A   Crawls.
B   Smiles socially.
C   Controls his bowel and bladder.
D   Sits unsupported.
E   Raises his head while prone.

1.9. A B C
By the age of 4 months most infants can roll over, have conjugate eye movements and can reach out and grab small objects. They do not sit with support until the age of 5 months and do not have incisor teeth until the age of 5–7 months.

1.10. A D
A normal full-term 6-month-old infant is able to sit with support and lift his head when prone, and support the upper trunk on extended arms. He shows no hand preference. The Moro reflex disappears by the age of 5 months. Most children will be able to fix and follow a moving face by the age of 6 weeks.

1.11. B C D
In achondroplasia and congenital hypothyroidism there is abnormality of the epiphyseal centres which results in diminution of linear growth of long bones. As a result the infantile body proportions (crown pubis/crown heel: 1.7/1) are maintained. In malnutrition there is delay in growth of ossification centres but there is no disturbance of epiphyseal growth. In Down syndrome the body proportions are normal. In osteogenesis imperfecta there may be shortening of limbs because of fractures.

1.12. A E
A 7-month-old infant is able to transfer an object from one hand to the other and is able to sit up. Toilet training is variable but is seldom achieved below the age of 2 years. Infants clap hands at the age of 8–9 months and are not distressed by the approach of strangers until the age of 7–8 months.

1.13. D
Both 5- and 7-month-old infants will smile and raise their head while prone, but will not crawl or be able to control their bowel and bladder. The 7-month-old would be able to sit unsupported whereas the 5-month-old would not.

1.14. Inability to do which of the following would be of concern in a baby of 9 months?

A   Sit unaided.
B   Use words with meaning.
C   Use pincer grip.
D   Put food in the mouth.
E   Change objects from one hand to the other.

1.15. Which of the following developmental attainments is/are appropriate for a child of 10 months?

A   Has good finger–thumb apposition with the left hand but uses a mild palmar grasp on the right.
B   Crawls symmetrically by dragging his extended legs behind, using his forearms.
C   Has a symmetrical forward parachute reaction.
D   Responds to noise but cannot localize the source.
E   Is mobile by shuffling along on his bottom in a sitting position.

1.16. Which of the following is/are true?

A   A 4-month-old infant is unlikely to produce vocal sounds other than crying.
B   An 8-month-old infant can hold his head steady in the sitting position.
C   A 6-month-old infant can be toilet-trained.
D   It is normal for a 9-month-old child to have no aversion to play in his urine or stool.
E   A 1-year-old child would be expected to give up a toy on request.

1.17. A 1-year-old child would be expected to

A   uncover an object (which was covered before he could grasp it).
B   grasp a raisin.
C   play simple ball games.
D   feed himself a biscuit.
E   put three words together.

1.14. A D E

More than 90% 9-month-old children can sit up unaided, put food in their mouth and transfer objects from one hand to the other. Pincer grip and words of meaning do not develop before the age of 10 months in most infants.

1.15. C E

A 10-month-old infant should have good finger–thumb apposition on both hands, crawl without dragging his legs, have a symmetrical parachute reaction, be able to localize sounds and move around by crawling or 'bottom shuffling'.

1.16. B D E

A 4-month-old infant would babble. Infants are able to hold their heads steady in the sitting position by the age of 3–4 months. Toilet training (as distinct from anticipation or 'reflex' training) cannot be achieved until the infant is able voluntarily to contract the anal sphincter and verbalize his needs. At the age of 9 months children have not developed the ability to distinguish between being clean and dirty. Children achieve the ability to give up a toy on request by the age of 8–9 months.

1.17. A B C D

At 9–10 months, infants can grasp a raisin, feed themselves with a biscuit and uncover an object covered in their presence. They can play simple ball games by the age of 1 year. They are not usually able to put three words together until the age of 2 years.

1.18. Ninety percent of children at 1 year would

A build a tower of three cubes.
B have a well developed pincer grip.
C give up a toy on request.
D walk without support.
E show stranger anxiety.

1.19. Which of the following behaviours are observed in a child at 12 months but not at 8 months of age?

A Stands alone well.
B Makes postural adjustments to dressing.
C Walks up steps.
D Finger–thumb grasp.
E Combines two words.

1.20. An infant aged 16 months was referred for assessment of suspected mental retardation. Which of the following findings is/are outside the range of normal?

A He does not scribble spontaneously with pencil on paper.   ⟹ 2 years
B He does not walk alone.
C 'Ma' and 'Dada' are the only words which are clearly recognizable.
D He is unable to build a tower of four cubes.
E He is unable to throw an object.

1.21. The majority of children at age 18 months are expected to be able to

A sit steadily on the floor unaided.
B say ten words.
C make a tower of three blocks when shown.
D find a toy under a cup.
E chew a biscuit.

1.18. B C E
More than 90% of children at 1 year would have a well-developed pincer grip (usually present at the age of 10 months), give up a toy on request and show anxiety towards strangers (usually present at 7–8 months). Most infants are unable to build a tower of three cubes before the age of 18 months and cannot walk without support until the age of 15 months.

1.19. A B D
In contrast to children at 8 months, children at 12 months are able to stand alone, make postural adjustments to dressing and have a well-developed pincer grip. They are unable to walk up steps or combine two words.

1.20. E
Children do not scribble until the age of 2 years. Not all children can walk alone by the age of 16 months. Many children at 16 months have a lot of jargon but may only have a few recognizable words. A child of 16 months would not be expected to make a tower of more than three cubes but can throw an object.

1.21. A B C D E
At the age of 18 months the majority of children have a vocabulary of 10 words and can make a tower of three blocks. They can sit up alone without support and chew a biscuit by the age of 9–10 months. They can find a toy under a cup at the age of 10 months.

1.22. A 1½ year old boy who walked at 10 months is a cause of concern and embarrassment to his parents because of unsightly bow legs (which are symmetrical) and marked in-toeing to which is attributed his frequent tipping and falling. His mother had similar problems which were treated by an osteopath, and now has no problems. Which of the following is/are correct?

A   The boy has an autosomal dominant condition.
B   The most likely diagnosis is vitamin D-resistant rickets.
C   Serum calcium and phosphorus levels will be normal.
D   Laboratory studies on vitamin D are not indicated.
E   The parents can be assured that the child requires no treatment.

1.23. Inability to do which of the following is a cause for concern in a 20-month child?

A   Speak in clear two to three word phrases.
B   Walk unaided.
C   Kick a ball.
D   Build a tower of eight blocks.
E   Cooperate with dressing.

1.24. By 2 years of age most children
A   are talking in three-word sentences.
B   are able to use a knife and fork.
C   know their surname.
D   can hop and skip.
E   can copy on paper crosses.

1.25. Most developmentally normal infants of 2 years
A   are able to kick a ball without falling.
B   can name three colours.
C   can ride a tricycle.
D   can build a tower of six blocks.
E   can use the past tense in speech.

1.22. C D E
Bow legs and in-toeing are normal in children up to the age of 2 years, after which they develop knock-knees which resolve by the age of 6 years. No investigations or treatment are necessary.

1.23. B E
More than 90% of children at the age of 20 months are able to walk unaided and cooperate with dressing. Ability to put eight blocks together is not achieved until the age of 30 months and the ability to put three words together is achieved at the age of 36 months. Ability to kick a ball is not achieved until the age of 24 months.

1.24. A
By the age of 2 years most children are able to put a subject, verb and object together, use a spoon (not knife and fork) and know their first name but not surname. They can draw crude crosses by the age of 3 years. Children cannot hop and skip until the age of 4 years.

1.25. A D
Children at 2 years can kick a ball without falling and build a tower of six blocks. They can name three colours by the age of 5 years and ride a tricycle at 3 years. They can use the past tense in speech at the age of 30–36 months.

1.26. Which of the following statements is/are true?

A Most infants can chew at 3 months.
B The normal respiratory rate of a 1-year-old child is between 20 and 30/min.
C A 2-year-old child is 'self-centred'.
D The average blood pressure of a 3-year-old child is 120/80 mmHg.
E A 5-year-old child is able to copy a circle.

1.27. Which of the following conditions is/are within the normal range of development at 4 years of age?

A Frequent faecal soiling.
B Frequent day wetting.
C Thumb sucking.
D Occasional masturbation.
E Night wetting.

1.28. A 5-year-old child should be able to

A draw a man (with body, head, etc.).
B identify four colours.
C copy a circle.
D count from 100 backwards.
E skip with alternate feet.

1.29. The majority of 6-year-old children would be expected to be able to

A hop on one foot.
B draw a recognizable picture of a man and include the head.
C define justice and honesty.
D identify their right and left arms.
E tie shoelaces.

1.30. Which of the following statements is/are true?

A An adolescent goitre is usually associated with hyperthyroidism.
B The early development of breast tissue in pubescent females is often unilateral.
C In girls the adolescent growth spurt follows the menarche by approximately 1 year.
D There has been a decrease in the age of menarche over the past century.
E The first sign of pubertal development in boys is growth of facial hair.

1.26. B C E

Infants are unable to carry the food to the back of the mouth with the tongue before the age of 4 months. At birth the normal respiratory rate is 40–60/min and it drops gradually to 20–30/min at the age of 1 year. By the age of 18 months the respiratory rate is between 15 and 25/min. Children at 2 years do not 'share' their possessions and tend to play 'in parallel' rather than participate in games. At birth the infant's blood pressure is 80/50 mmHg and it progressively increases throughout life. Adult values (120/80 mmHg) are not reached until the age of 16 years. Most children are able to copy a circle by the age of 5 years.

1.27. C D E

Thumb sucking, occasional masturbation and night wetting are normal for a child of 4 years. Most children are dry by day and do not have faecal soiling by this age.

1.28. A B C E

A 5-year-old child will be able to draw a man (with body, head and four or five parts), identify four colours, copy a circle, skip and be able to count up to ten.

1.29. A B D E

Children can hop on one foot at the age of 5 years, draw a recognizable picture of a man with two to four parts other than the head at the age of 4 years, identify right and left arms and tie their shoelaces at the age of 6 years. They do not conceptualize abstract terms such as justice and honesty until the age of 8–10 years.

1.30. B D

Breast development is usually asymmetrical and may cause anxiety to prepubescent girls. The adolescent growth spurt occurs prior to menarche. The decrease in the age of menarche is thought to be due to better nutrition. The first sign of pubertal development in boys is the increase in size of the testes. Adolescent goitres are euthyroid.

1.31. Which of the following problems are more likely to be found in adolescents than in children under 12 years old?
A   Recurrent abdominal pain.
B   Crohn's disease.
C   Intussusception.
D   Conduct disorder.
E   Acne.

1.32. Which of the following statements about puberty is/are correct?
A   The peak height velocity usually occurs following the onset of menstruation in girls.
B   There is an increase in androgen secretion at puberty in girls.
C   The pituitary hormone which stimulates hormonal activity by the gonads is the same in both sexes.
D   The average peak height velocity occurs at an earlier age in girls than in boys.
E   The average peak height velocity is less in girls than in boys.

1.33. Which of the following statements is/are true of sexual development at puberty?
A   Sexual maturation is more closely correlated with bone maturation than with chronological age.
B   Girls mature earlier than boys.
C   Testicular enlargement is the first sign of puberty in boys.
D   Breast hypertrophy is rare (less than 10%) in boys at puberty.
E   During the first year following menarche, the menstrual periods of most girls are anovulatory.

1.34. Which of the following has/have an increased incidence in adolescence?
A   Thyrotoxicosis.
B   Acne vulgaris.
C   Peptic ulceration.
D   Anorexia nervosa.
E   Scoliosis.

1.31. B D E
Recurrent abdominal pains are more likely to occur in children below the age of 12. Intussusception most commonly occurs in infants aged 6–9 months. Crohn's disease, conduct disorder and acne are more likely to be found in adolescents than in children under 12 years old.

1.32. B C D E
The peak height velocity in girls occurs at the onset of puberty, which is well before the onset of menstruation. Increased androgen secretion by the adrenal gland is responsible for the development of pubic and axillary hair in girls as well as in boys. Follicle-stimulating hormone (FSH) stimulates the production of testosterone and oestrogen. The peak height velocity in girls occurs at 12–14 years, compared with 12.5–15 years in boys. However, the average peak height velocity is less in girls than in boys because of the earlier onset of their growth spurt.

1.33. A B C E
Bone and sexual maturation are both under the control of androgens and may not have any correlation with chronological age. Girls mature an average of 1–2 years earlier than boys. Testicular enlargement is the first sign of puberty in boys. Breast hypertrophy is common in boys. Menstrual periods are anovulatory in the first year after menarche in most girls.

1.34. A B D E
The peak incidence of thyrotoxicosis occurs in adolescence. At puberty increased levels of androgens cause an increase in size and secretions of sebaceous follicles, resulting in acne. Anorexia nervosa and scoliosis have their onset in early puberty and have an increased incidence in girls. There is no evidence for an increased incidence of peptic ulceration at puberty.

1.35. Which of the following statements is/are correct?

A   Testicular volume of 3 ml is within normal limits for Tanner stage IV penile and pubic hair development.

B   Asymmetrical breast development can be normal in a 13-year-old girl.

C   A 4-year-old boy with tall stature, large penis and pubic hair is likely to have congenital adrenal hyperplasia.

D   Precocious sexual development with normal bone age is most likely to represent idiopathic sexual precocity.

E   At a bone age of 15, a boy is unlikely to grow more than 5 cm irrespective of treatment.

1.36. A 10-month-old male child who at 5 months was on the 50th percentile for height, weight and head circumference is now still on the 50th percentile for height and weight but is above the 97th percentile for head circumference. Which of the following statements is/are true?

A   It is not of concern if either parent's head circumference is on or above the 97th percentile.

B   The parents can be reassured as the head circumference is within normal range.

C   He ought to be reviewed in 6 months.

D   The head circumference should be measured again and checked.

E   The child should be referred for specialist assessment.

1.37. Which of the following statements is/are true of a child aged 8 months whose length lies on the 10th percentile and whose head circumference lies on the 10th percentile?

A   He is abnormally short and should be investigated.

B   He is likely to be normal.

C   He is suffering from microcephaly.

D   He is at least as long as 10 in every 100 children of his age.

E   He is failing to thrive.

1.38. Gynaecomastia in boys is significantly associated with

A   obesity.

B   Klinefelter's syndrome.

C   Noonan's syndrome.

D   cirrhosis of the liver.

E   feminizing tumour of the adrenals.

1.35. B C E

Tanner stage IV penile and pubic hair development indicates onset of puberty. At this stage the testicular size is more than 4 ml. Asymmetrical breast development is normal in both sexes. Congenital adrenal hyperplasia results in precocious puberty. As fusion of tibial and fibular epiphyses is complete in boys by the age of 16 years, further significant increase in height is unlikely. Sexual precosity is accompanied by an increase in bone age.

1.36. D E

Children may have large heads because their parents' head sizes are large. Even though the head circumference is normal for some children, it is abnormal for this child as it has crossed centiles while the weight and height have remained on the same centiles. The head circumference should be measured again to ensure that the measurement is correct. If it is correct, specialist referral is indicated. Frequent review (fortnightly or monthly) is mandatory.

1.37. B D

As this child's head circumference and length fall on the same centiles the child does not require any investigations for 'short stature'. The child's head circumference is normal for his length. The 10th percentile means that 10% of the children are the same length or shorter than this child. Without knowing the weight of the child it is incorrect to say that he is 'failing to thrive'.

1.38. B D E

Obesity and Noonan's syndrome are not associated with gynaecomastia. In Klinefelter's syndrome there is deficiency of androgen and gynaecomastia. Oestrogens are responsible for gynaecomastia in cirrhosis of the liver (failure of metabolism of oestrogens) and in feminizing tumour of the adrenals (excessive oestrogen production by the adrenal gland).

1.39. Which of the following statements is/are true of brain growth?

A   There is a period of rapid postnatal growth of the cerebellum during the first year of life.

B   The brain is 50% of the adult size at 5 years of age.

C   There is no growth due to an increase in cell number after birth.

D   There is little growth as a result of an increase in number of neurones after 12 months postnatal age.

E   Cell number and cell connections increase in parallel during growth of the brain.

1.40. Which of the following statements is/are true of skeletal growth?

A   The change from infantile to mature facial proportions is due to the more rapid growth of the upper part of the facial skeleton than of the lower part.

B   Elongation of the long bones in childhood and adolescence occurs mainly at the primary ossification centres.

C   Relative to ossified bone, the amount of cartilage in bone increases with maturity.

D   High doses of androgens accelerate bone maturation (e.g. epiphyseal fusion) more rapidly than linear growth.

E   The lower femoral epiphyses are evident on X-ray before the upper femoral epiphyses.

1.41. Skeletal proportions are normal in

A   pituitary dwarfism.

B   achondroplasia.

C   delayed adolescence.

D   congenital hypothyroidism.

E   emotional deprivation.

1.42. The anterior fontanelle

A   usually closes by 3 months of age.

B   is rarely pulsatile.

C   marks the junction of the sagittal and coronal sutures.

D   may not bulge in the presence of meningitis.

E   is usually smaller than the posterior fontanelle

1.39. A D

During the first year of life the cerebellum grows rapidly. The brain is almost adult size by the age of 5 years. The brain of the term infant contains the full adult component of neurones. In the first year brain size increases as a result of myelination, elaboration of neuronal processes (both neurones and dendrites) and increase in glial cells. Subsequently it is mainly due to elaboration of neuronal processes.

1.40. D E

The mandible grows faster than the rest of the face at puberty. Elongation of long bones occurs both at primary and secondary ossification centres. With maturity the cartilage is replaced by ossified bone. Androgens accelerate bone maturation and stimulate osteogenesis, which results in epiphyseal fusion and ultimate diminution of linear growth. The lower femoral epiphysis is present at birth whereas the upper femoral epiphysis appears in the first year of life.

1.41. A C E

In achondroplasia and congenital hypothyroidism the limbs grow slowly because of epiphyseal dysplasia. In delayed adolescence growth of long bones continues for a longer period, resulting in normal body proportions. In pituitary dwarfism and emotional deprivation there is lack of growth hormone and body proportions remain normal.

1.42. C D

The anterior fontanelle usually closes between 9 and 18 months. It is pulsatile and marks the junction of the sagittal and coronal sutures. It is larger than the posterior fontanelle. Although a bulging fontanelle is seen in meningitis, it may not be present in newborn infants and infants suffering from dehydration.

1.43. Delayed eruption of teeth can occur in
A   rickets.
B   severe neonatal hyperbilirubinaemia.
C   hypothyroidism.
D   cleidocranial dysostosis.
E   ectodermal dysplasia.

1.44. Which of the following statements concerning teething is/are correct?
A   A 1-year-old infant is likely to have six to eight deciduous teeth.
B   The first deciduous tooth to erupt is an upper central incisor.
C   There are 20 deciduous teeth.
D   One of the first permanent teeth to erupt is a lower central incisor.
E   Calcification of the first permanent molars begins at birth in a full-term infant.

1.45. Retardation of bone age is a recognized feature of
A   obesity.
B   malabsorption.
C   congenital adrenal cortical hyperplasia.
D   isolated growth hormone deficiency.
E   psychosocial deprivation.

1.46. Teething is a recognized cause of
A   diarrhoea.
B   seizures.
C   salivation with lip dribbling.
D   irritability.
E   anaemia.

1.47. During growth and development
A   thyroid hormone plays an essential part in the maturation of tissues.
B   'bone age' correlates more closely with 'height age' than with 'weight age'.
C   the testes are usually in the scrotum by the end of the fourth month of fetal life.
D   the earliest sign of puberty in a boy is enlargement of the testes.
E   menarche occurs with onset of breast development at puberty.

1.43. A C D
Delayed eruption of the teeth occurs in hypothyroidism, rickets and cleido-cranial dysostosis. Severe neonatal hyperbilirubinaemia causes blue to black discolouration of teeth. In ectodermal dysplasia, the teeth are totally or partially absent.

1.44. A C D E
There is great variability in dental eruption. By the age of 1 year most children will have six to eight teeth. Usually the first tooth to erupt is a lower central incisor. There are 20 deciduous teeth. The first permanent tooth to erupt is the first molar or lower central incisor; this occurs at 6–7 years of age. Calcification of the first permanent molar begins at birth in a term infant.

1.45. B D E
Bone age is retarded in malabsorption, growth hormone deficiency and psychosocial deprivation. It is accelerated in obesity and in congenital adrenal cortical hyperplasia. In the latter this is due to increased androgen production.

1.46. C D
Teething has been assumed to be the cause of many infantile problems (including fever, diarrhoea, fits) because of its chance association with those conditions. Irritability and salivation with dribbling are due to the pain associated with eruption of the teeth.

1.47. A B D
Thyroid hormone plays an important part in maturation of tissues in periods of rapid growth. Bone age correlates more closely with height age than with weight age. The testes are in the scrotum by 32–34 weeks' gestation. The earliest sign of puberty in a boy is enlargement of the testes. The onset of menarche occurs much later than breast development at puberty.

1.48. Compared with girls, boys

A have a higher infant mortality.
B exhibit the adolescent growth spurt earlier.
C are more likely to have hereditary microspherocytosis.
D are more likely to be accidentally drowned.
E pass their milestones of infant development earlier.

1.49. Development of speech in an infant can be delayed by

A late eruption of teeth.
B cleft lip.
C emotional deprivation.
D enlarged adenoids.
E deafness.

1.50. Which of the following statements is/are correct?

A Isolated delay in speech development is an indication for a hearing test.
B Presence of babbling does not exclude deafness.
C Tongue tie is a common cause of delayed speech.
D Girls tend to speak at an earlier age than boys.
E Delay in speech development is often familial.

1.51. A child with bilateral cleft lip and palate is more likely to have which of the following speech and/or language problems?

A Weak pressure on consonants.
B High-pitched voice.
C Stuttering.
D Delayed language development.
E Nasal air escape during speech.

1.52. A congenitally deaf but intelligent child of 4 years would show which of the following?

A If he can speak his voice will have metallic and monotonous quality.
B Communication by gesture.
C Purposeless play.
D Frustration tantrums.
E Clumsiness and incoordination.

1.48. A D
Boys have a higher mortality than girls at all ages. They exhibit the adolescent growth spurt later and are more likely to be accidentally drowned. The inheritance of microspherocytosis is autosomal dominant and there is no difference in incidence between the two sexes. The infant developmental milestones are similar in both sexes.

1.49. C E
Late speech can result from emotional deprivation and deafness. It has no relationship to late eruption of teeth or cleft lip. Enlarged adenoids might distort speech and cause nasal intonation.

1.50. A B D E
Isolated delay in speech development may be due to loss of hearing. Babbling occurs irrespective of hearing but does not progress to recognizable speech in deaf children. Tongue tie does not cause delayed speech though it may cause indistinct speech. Girls tend to speak at an earlier age than boys. Delay in speech development is often familial.

1.51. A E
Children with bilateral cleft lip and palate have problems with pronunciation because of nasal air escape during speech. Their voice is not high-pitched and they do not have stuttering.

1.52. A B D
A congenitally deaf but intelligent child of 4 years would not have purposeless play or show clumsiness and incoordination. If he speaks at all he would have a monotonous voice. He communicates by gesture and is frustrated because of his inability to communicate.

1.53. Delay in language development is common in

A   autism.
B   deafness.
C   elective mutism.
D   twins.
E   gross emotional deprivation.

1.54. In normal language development

A   babbling ceases at 6–9 months.
B   vocabulary at 2 years usually comprises about 25–30 words.
C   construction of short sentences is achieved by one year.
D   pronouns are used from 18 months.
E   construction of complex sentences is achieved by 4 years.

1.55. If a 3-year-old male child is neither speaking clearly nor making sentences

A   he should have his hearing tested.
B   his speech function could be within normal limits.
C   the child has a 90% chance of being mentally retarded.
D   he should not attend a day-care centre until his speech is improved.
E   the amount of stimulation to speak should be assessed.

1.53. A B D E
Delay in language development is a feature of autism and gross emotional deprivation. Deafness results in delay in language development because of inability to hear. Twins tend to speak later than singletons because they can communicate with each other and have less need to speak. In elective mutism language development is not delayed.

1.54. D E
Babbling persists until at least the age of 12 months. By the age of 18 months a child has a vocabulary of 50 words. Construction of short sentences (subject, verb, object) is not achieved till the age of 2 years. Children begin to refer to self with the pronoun 'I' or 'me' by the age of 15 months. By 4 years children are able to construct complex sentences, e.g. relative clauses.

1.55. A B E
Hearing loss is a common cause of unclear speech as the child does not hear the words correctly. Children who have things done for them or can have their needs met by pointing to things generally do not speak in sentences. Such children benefit from the stimulation provided at a day-care centre. Delay in speech may be the presenting symptom of mental retardation; however, many 3-year-old normal children will not have clear speech.

2 Nutrition

2.1. Breast milk production is likely to be increased by
A   extra water in the mother's diet.
B   a strongly sucking infant.
C   extra milk in the mother's diet.
D   administration of stilboestrol.
E   maximal emptying of the breasts.

2.2. Which of the following statements is/are correct about the let-down reflex?
A   Prolonged rapid shallow sucking by the infant indicates efficient let-down.
B   Delay in let-down is caused by stress in the mother.
C   A deep rhythmical suck/swallow pattern with short pauses during feeding indicates efficient let-down.
D   The let-down reflex is facilitated by the baby sucking.
E   The let-down reflex is facilitated by oxytocin.

2.3. The mother of a newborn infant presents with a red, hot, hard and painful segment in the upper outer quadrant of her left breast accompanied with rigors. Her temperature is 38°C. Which of the following statements is/are correct?
A   The most likely diagnosis is breast engorgement.
B   The mother should be treated with amoxicillin and flucloxacillin.
C   Until resolution of the problem, the breast milk will need to be discarded as it is infected.
D   Incomplete emptying of the breast has contributed to the problem.
E   Breast feeding should be encouraged as cessation will predispose to abscess.

2.4. Human colostrum compared with mature human milk
A   has a higher fat content.
B   has fewer cellular elements.
C   is richer in secretory IgA.
D   contains more protein.
E   has a lower water content.

2.1. B E
Breast milk production is increased by regular and complete emptying of breast manually or a strongly sucking infant. Extra water or milk in the diet or stilboestrol do not increase breast milk production.

2.2. B C D E
The let-down reflex is inhibited by stress. It is stimulated by oxytocin and the sight or cry of the infant. With an efficient let-down reflex the infant sucks rhythmically, alternating swallowing with pauses. On the other hand with a poor let-down reflex, the infant has prolonged rapid shallow sucking.

2.3. B D E
Unlike breast engorgement, breast infection presents with localized tenderness and induration as it is due to invasion of organisms via a lactiferous duct to a secretory lobule. In such cases the lobule should be kept empty in order to prevent abscess formation. The mother needs treatment with antibiotics effective against *Staphylococcus aureus, E. coli* and streptococci. Although the milk contains organisms, the infants who consume the milk do not become ill.

2.4. C D
The fat content of human milk is slightly higher than that of colostrum, which is richer in secretory IgA and contains more protein. Colostrum has more cellular elements. The water content of the two milks is approximately the same.

2.5. Compared with human milk, pasteurized cows' milk has higher content of

A calories.
B water.
C carbohydrates.
D electrolytes.
E iron.

2.6. Compared with human milk, cows' milk contains more

A protein.
B phosphate.
C vitamin K.
D lactose.
E sodium.

2.7. Cows' milk protein intolerance (allergy) can

A cause vomiting.
B present with blood streaking of stools.
C result in failure to thrive.
D be treated with lactose-free formulas.
E occur in exclusively breast-fed infants.

2.8. Which of the following may occur in a 2-week-old infant who has been fed on whole cows' milk?

A An elevated blood urea nitrogen.
B Dehydration.
C Convulsions.
D Elevated serum sodium.
E Low serum potassium.

2.9. Which of the following statements regarding infant feeding is/are correct?

A The daily fluid volume requirements per kilogram of preterm babies are higher than those of full-term infants.
B The fluid requirements of small-for-dates infants per kilogram are higher than those of infants who are appropriate for gestation.
C Fat should provide 10–15% of an infant's caloric intake.
D Fully breast-fed infants do not develop infantile eczema.
E The sugar of breast milk is the same sugar as in cows' milk.

2.5. D
The caloric and water content of human and cows' milk is approximately the same. The carbohydrate and iron content of human milk is greater than that of cows' milk. Cows' milk contains three to four times the electrolyte content of human milk.

2.6. A B C E
Compared with human milk, cows' milk contains approximately twice as much protein, six times the amount of phosphate, four times the amount of vitamin K and three times the amount of sodium. The lactose content of human milk is approximately twice that of cows' milk.

2.7. A B C E
Cows' milk protein intolerance can cause vomiting and diarrohoea (which results in failure to thrive) and faecal blood loss due to colitis. It has been reported in fully breast-fed infants since the protein can enter breast-milk from the mother's ingested cows' milk. It can be successfully treated with soya formulas (but not lactose-free cows' milk formulas) though such infants are prone to develop soya milk protein intolerance (allergy) as well.

2.8. A B C D
Whole cows' milk has higher content of protein, phosphorus and electrolytes than human milk. As the kidney of a 2-week-old infant is unable to handle this extra load, as well as a result of metabolism of the extra protein, this results in raised blood urea nitrogen and raised serum sodium which cause osmotic diuresis resulting in dehydration. The high phosphorus level prevents absorption of calcium from the gut leading to low serum calcium, which may present with convulsions. Serum potassium is normal or raised.

2.9. A B E
The fluid requirements of preterm infants and small-for-dates infants are 180–200 ml/kg compared with 150 ml/kg for full-term infants who are appropriate for gestation because they have greater loss of fluid (increase of surface area relative to weight and respiratory rate). Fats provide about one-third of the infant's caloric intake. Breast feeding does not provide protection against infantile eczema. The sugar in both breast and cows' milk is lactose.

2.10. For a full-term exclusively breast-fed thriving baby, which of the following feeding practices is/are recommended?

A   Iron supplementation from the age of 2 months.
B   Fluoride supplementation of the mother from delivery.
C   Vitamin C supplementation from the age of 2 months.
D   Commencement of solids at about 4 months.
E   Weaning to cows' milk at about 6 months.

2.11. Which of the following statements is/are true?

A   Xerophthalmia in a 3-year-old child is pathognomonic of vitamin A deficiency.
B   Vitamin A overdose can cause raised intracranial pressure.
C   Scurvy is rare in breast-fed infants.
D   Vitamin D deficiency in infants can present with seizures.
E   Vitamin E deficiency predisposes to haemolysis.

2.12. Which of the following statements concerning vitamins is/are true?

A   Mega-doses of vitamin A have been shown to be toxic.
B   Vitamin D_3 (cholecalciferol) is a naturally occurring vitamin in fish oils.
C   Vitamin C is destroyed during cooking.
D   Babies fed on goats' milk require supplements of folic acid.
E   Cows' milk contains less vitamin K than human milk.

2.13. Which of the following statements is/are true about vitamin C?

A   It is essential for the formation of collagen.
B   It corrects transient tyrosinaemia in low-birth-weight infants.
C   Formula-fed babies require vitamin C supplementation.
D   Scorbutic rosary (due to vitamin C deficiency) is indistinguishable from rachitic rosary.
E   Paucity of limb movements may be a presenting symptom of vitamin C deficiency.

2.10. D
Full-term infants do not need iron supplementation until the age of 4–6 months as they accumulate adequate amounts of iron in the last trimester of pregnancy. Fluoride does not appear in adequate quantities in breast milk. There is an adequate amount of vitamin C in breast milk. Solids are started at about age 4 months so that the infant is on adequate solids by the age of 6 months. Whole cows' milk can cause gastrointestinal bleeding and is not recommended until after the age of 1 year.

2.11. A B C D E
Xerophthalmia (dryness of conjunctiva and cornea) is due to vitamin A deficiency. Vitamin A overdose causes raised intracranial pressure. There are adequate amounts of vitamin C in breast milk. Vitamin D deficiency in infants results in hypocalcaemia and tetany as well as seizures. Vitamin E deficiency results in haemolysis due to instability of the red cell membrane.

2.12. A C D
Excess vitamin A causes anorexia, slow growth, drying and cracking of the skin, enlargement of liver and spleen, swelling and pain of long bones, bone fragility and increased intracranial pressure. Vitamin D_3 is activated 7-dehydrocholesterol, which is normally present in human skin. Vitamin C is easily oxidized; this is accelerated by heat, light, alkali and oxidative enzymes. Goats' milk is deficient in folic acid. Cows' milk contains four times more vitamin K than human milk.

2.13. A B C E
Vitamin C is essential for the formation of collagen. It corrects the transient tyrosinaemia in low-birth-weight infants. It is destroyed during processing of milk formulae. Its deficiency results in irritability and pain in the limbs due to periosteal haemorrhage, which presents as pseudoparalysis. Scorbutic rosary is due to dislocation of costochondral junctions resulting in angulation, which is easily distinguishable from rachitic rosary (widened epiphysis).

2.14. A 7-month-old infant is admitted with seizures and found to have a serum calcium of 1.5 mmol/l, phosphorus 1.0 mmol/l and elevated alkaline phosphatase of 600. Which of the following statements is/are true?
A Neurological sequelae are common.
B Vitamin D therapy is required.
C Concomitant aminoaciduria indicates renal tubular disease.
D Vitamin B_{12} deficiency needs to be ruled out.
E Congenital hypothyroidism is a likely diagnosis.

2.15. Craniotabes is significantly associated with
A rickets.
B osteogenesis imperfecta.
C thalassaemia minor.
D lacunar skull.
E prematurity.

2.16. If the intake of calories in an infant is chronically insufficient in quantity but with a reasonable proportion derived from protein
A he will have good subcutaneous fat stores but inadequate muscle bulk.
B replacement of some of the carbohydrate with protein will make little difference to the clinical state of the child.
C head growth will be markedly decreased for age.
D weight will be decreased for age.
E the serum protein will usually be decreased.

2.17. Biochemical abnormalities in kwashiorkor include
A hypernatraemia.
B aminoaciduria.
C lactase deficiency.
D low serum albumin.
E potassium deficiency.

2.14. B

A low serum calcium and phosphorus with a high serum alkaline phosphotase indicates that the infant has vitamin D-deficient rickets with seizures. Such infants have aminoaciduria and do not have neurological sequelae. There is no indication that the infant has vitamin B_{12} deficiency or thyroid disease.

2.15. A B E

In rickets and prematurity the skull is soft because of inadequate calcification. In osteogenesis imperfecta there is deficiency of bone matrix. In lacunar skull there are defects in the vault in the form of depressions or 'holes' extending to the outer surface of the skull, mainly in the frontal or parietal regions. There is no softening of the skull in thalassaemia minor.

2.16. B D

In the presence of insufficient caloric intake, there is loss of subcutaneous fat tissue and weight. There is little (if any) disturbance of head growth. The serum protein will be maintained within normal values by breakdown of muscle tissue. As long as the total calories are inadequate the clinical state will remain unchanged irrespective of whether the patient eats carbohydrate or protein.

2.17. B C D E

Low serum albumin which results in oedema is the characteristic feature of kwashiorkor. Serum sodium is low or normal. Aminoaciduria results from disturbed renal function. Lactase deficiency is a result of a decrease in intestinal enzymes due to subtotal villous atrophy. Potassium and magnesium deficiencies are common.

2.18. Which of the following statements is/are true of severe protein–calorie malnutrition?

A There will be normal subcutaneous fat stores but inadequate muscle bulk.

B Replacement of some of the carbohydrate with protein will make little difference to the clinical state.

C Total body water as percentage of body weight will be increased.

D The serum proteins will usually be markedly decreased.

E Total body potassium will be decreased.

2.19. Which of the following statements about vitamin K is/are correct?

A Cord blood levels are lower than maternal blood.

B Excess causes thrombosis.

C Oral vitamin K at birth is adequate prophylaxis for late haemorrhagic disease.

D Adequate amounts are present in breast milk.

E Intramuscular injection has been demonstrated conclusively to increase the incidence of childhood malignancy.

2.20. Failure to thrive

A is most commonly due to an organic cause.

B is most commonly due to lack of calories.

C usually requires a battery of laboratory tests to determine the cause.

D always requires documentation of caloric intake so that underfeeding due to error or ignorance is ruled out.

E responds to feeding if the cause is organic.

2.21. A child with moderate malnutrition following a chronic diarrhoeal illness is likely to have

A a greater fall off in length centile than of head circumference centile.

B muscle hypotonia.

C loss of turgor.

D hyperkalaemia.

E iron deficiency anaemia.

2.18. B C E

In protein–calorie malnutrition there is deficiency of calories which results in loss of subcutaneous fat. As the total calories remain unchanged, the protein that replaces carbohydrate will be used up to meet the caloric needs. The total body water as percentage of body weight increases as the lean body weight is proportionately increased. Unlike protein malnutrition, in protein–calorie malnutrition the serum proteins are maintained because muscle tissue is being broken down to meet the caloric needs which supplies part of the protein. Total body potassium is decreased because of decrease in muscle tissue.

2.19. A

Vitamin K crosses the placenta poorly. As a result maternal plasma vitamin K levels are higher than cord blood levels. Large doses of synthetic vitamin K have been reported to cause haemolysis, jaundice and kernicterus in premature infants. Late haemorrhagic disease occurs almost exclusively in breast-fed infants given no vitamin K or a single oral dose at birth, though it may also occur in infants given intramuscular vitamin K. Breast milk fails to supply the recommended daily allowance (RDA) of vitamin K to infants. Although one report indicated that intramuscular vitamin K increased the incidence of childhood malignancy, subsequent studies have failed to confirm the association.

2.20. B D

Unless obvious, organic causes of failure to thrive are uncommon. Even in developed countries the most common cause of failure to thrive is lack of calories; this is not necessarily due to inadequate availability of food, hence documentation of caloric intake is important. If the cause is organic it will not respond to feeding alone.

2.21. A B E

In malnutrition the growth pattern that is most affected is weight followed by length and then head circumference. Muscle hypotonia results. Iron deficiency anaemia is a result of lack of absorption. Although there is low total body potassium, serum potassium is usually normal. Dehydration (loss of skin turgor) is not a prominent feature in chronic diarrhoeal illness.

2.22. Which of the following statements is/are true?

A The calorie intake of aerated drinks, fruit juices and cordials is too small to account for excessive weight gain.

B Obese children tend to eat more rapidly than their healthy peers.

C Obese children are less discriminating in their choice of foods.

D Sleep apnoea is frequently observed among excessively obese children.

E Obese children are more accident prone than their peers.

2.23. Which of the following is typical of an obese 8-year-old boy?

A Greater than average height.

B Normal bone age.

C Normal size external genitalia.

D Unusual happy temperament.

E Delayed puberty.

2.24. Which of the following statements is/are true about juvenile obesity?

A Inactivity of children plays a causal role.

B The child of an obese parent has an increased chance of being obese.

C There is some degree of insulin resistance.

D It is associated with greater than average height.

E In developed countries there is a higher incidence in lower than in middle and upper socio-economic class persons.

2.25. A 2-year-old girl is brought to see you with the complaint that she eats 'nothing'. The child is active and appears well. She weighs 11.5 kg (50th percentile) and her height is 90 cm (75th percentile). Physical examination reveals no abnormality. Which of the following statements is/are correct with regard to the management of this child?

A She should be given a tonic.

B She should be forced to eat.

C She should be investigated for urinary tract problems.

D Parents should be reassured that there is nothing wrong with her.

E Parents should stop fussing about her eating.

2.22. B C D E
Aerated drinks, fruit juices and cordials contain large amounts of disaccharides and sorbitol. Obese children do not adequately chew their food and eat rapidly as a result. Their appetite is not satisfied and they become less discriminating in their choice of food. They are prone to sleep apnoea because of carbon dioxide narcosis due to hypoventilation. The incidence of accidents is increased in obese children.

2.23. A C
Obesity tends to be associated with accelerated growth (including height, bone age and puberty). The external genitalia, though normal, appear to be small because of the excess amount of fat in the pubic region. The temperament is no different from other children of their age, though they may be depressed because of teasing.

2.24. A B D E
Obese children tend to be inactive which further aggravates the problem. Epidemiological studies have shown there is an increased familial incidence and a higher incidence in lower than in middle or upper socio-economic classes in developed countries. Obesity tends to increase height velocity. There is no evidence that there is any insulin resistance in obesity.

2.25. D E
The height and weight of this child suggest that she is growing normally. Therefore she does not need any investigations or treatment. Parents need reassurance and should be advised not to fuss.

3 Genetics and metabolic disorders

3.1. Concerning spontaneous early abortions (first trimester), which of the following statements is/are true?

A   The incidence of chromosome abnormalities in the abortuses is between 5 and 15%.

B   Trisomy 21 is the most frequent single chromosome abnormality in the abortuses.

C   The incidence of 45,X karyotype in the abortuses is approximately the same as in the liveborn population.

D   There is an increased incidence of abnormal karyotype in parents who have had frequent (more than four) spontaneous miscarriages.

E   Trisomy in an abortus implies an increased risk for younger mothers that a subsequent pregnancy would also be trisomic.

3.2. Fred and his wife have had three miscarriages as well as one healthy offspring. Fred is shown to be a carrier of a balanced reciprocal translocation between chromosomes 3 and 22-t(3:22)(q21;q11). In advising Fred and his family about this finding which statement(s) is/are true?

A   If Fred's parents are tested one of them will be shown to carry the same translocation.

B   In a subsequent pregnancy prenatal diagnosis would not be possible until midtrimester (18–20 weeks).

C   If Fred's sister and brother are both shown to be carriers the risk for abnormal offspring is greater for the sister's offspring.

D   The most likely consequence of abnormal segregation is miscarriage.

E   The couple's normal offspring should be offered genetic counselling.

3.3. Which of the following have been shown to be associated with an increased risk of congenital malformations?

A   Maternal smoking.

B   Maternal diabetes.

C   Maternal ingestion of alcohol.

D   Maternal ingestion of phenytoin.

E   Maternal ingestion of salicylates.

3.1. D E

Routine investigations of spontaneous abortions in the first trimester have shown that at least 50% have chromosome abnormalities and that 45,X is the most frequent single chromosome abnormality. The vast majority (about 99%) of 45,X fetuses are aborted spontaneously. The incidence of chromosome abnormality (specifically balanced translocations and other rearrangements) is approximately 6% in parents who have had more than three spontaneous miscarriages. Trisomy in an abortus increases the likelihood that trisomy may occur in a subsequent pregnancy if the mother is less than 35. Over this age there is probably no increase in risk above that for other women of the same age.

3.2. C D E

Reciprocal translocations are frequently found to be *de novo*, i.e. not present in either parent. Prenatal diagnosis is possible by chorionic villus sampling (CVS) at 10 weeks as well as by amniocentesis in midtrimester (15–17 weeks). Female translocation carriers are at greater risk of abnormal offspring than are male carriers. Most abnormal segregants from reciprocal translocations are sufficiently unbalanced to result in spontaneous pregnancy loss, but the proportion varies with the specific translocation. If the parent has a balanced rearrangement there is a risk that the offspring could be unbalanced but viable. Mental retardation and or malformation can result. If one of his parents is shown to carry the translocation then the normal offspring could also be a balanced carrier who would be at risk of abnormal pregnancy outcome.

3.3. B C D

Maternal diabetes increases the risk of congenital heart disease and spinal malformations. Optimal control minimizes this risk. Excessive maternal ingestion of alcohol increases the risk of microcephaly, growth retardation, intellectual deficit and facial dysmorphism. Maternal ingestion of phenytoin is also associated with a syndrome of low birth weight, mental retardation, unusual facies and congenital heart defect. The incidence of cleft lip and palate is increased. The ingestion of salicylates during pregnancy is not considered to have any teratogenic effect and neither is maternal smoking.

3.4. Which of the following increase the risk of congenital anomalies?

A   Maternal pre-eclampsia.

B   Isotretinoin (Roaccutane) ingestion during pregnancy.

C   As few as three chest X-rays in early pregnancy.

D   Maternal hyperthermia of more than 2°C above normal body temperature.

E   Oral contraceptives in the first 6 weeks of pregnancy.

3.5. For which of the following conditions is prenatal diagnosis possible by high resolution ultrasound scanning prior to 20 weeks' gestation?

A   Renal agenesis.

B   Anencephaly.

C   Down syndrome.

D   Fetal sex.

E   Cystic fibrosis.

3.6. In which of the following circumstances can prenatal diagnosis be offered based on analysis of tissue obtained from chorionic villus sampling alone?

A   A second pregnancy of a mother with no previous family history who has had a previous child with Duchenne muscular dystrophy (DMD) due to a deletion in the dystrophin gene.

B   Third pregnancy of a mother over 40 whose previous children have been clinically normal but who is concerned about the risks of chromosomal abnormality.

C   Second pregnancy of a mother aged 26, the previous child having cleft palate.

D   Third pregnancy of a mother who has had a previous child with cystic fibrosis (CF) who has since died without DNA investigations and the parents have not been studied.

E   The second pregnancy of a mother who has had a previous child affected with beta thalassaemia and no DNA testing of the family has been done.

3.4. B D

Vitamin A analogues such as isotretinoin (Roaccutane) and etretinate (Tigason), which are used to treat severe acne, are contraindicated in pregnancy because they are potent teratogens. X-rays during pregnancy are a common cause for concern, but the radiation level to which the fetus is exposed from a small number of standard radiological procedures, such as standard X-rays, is well below that associated with birth defects such as microcephaly. Certain formulations of oral contraceptives have been implicated in masculinization of female fetuses but this effect does not occur until 8 weeks of gestation onwards. Hyperthermia increases the risk of congenital malformations. Maternal pre-eclampsia does not cause congenital anomalies, although it may be associated with them.

3.5. A B D

Renal agenesis can be diagnosed by ultrasound before 20 weeks, as can almost all neural tube defects, particularly anencephaly. Down syndrome can only be reliably detected by karyotype analysis. Although fetal genitalia can frequently be visualized from 16 weeks' gestation onwards this would not be adequate for fetal sexing for a serious genetic condition. The diagnosis of cystic fibrosis by ultrasound alone is not possible.

3.6. A B

A woman who has had one previous child with DMD may or may not be a carrier. The first step would be to attempt to ascertain her carrier status, though this is not always possible. Prenatal diagnosis can be offered if the deletion in the affected boy is known (as in this case) or where there is a family history of other affected individuals and linkage information (indirect DNA testing) can be utilized. This is not always possible. A 40-year-old woman, no matter how many normal children she has had previously, has a 1 in 112 risk of a liveborn infant with Down syndrome and a 1 in 64 of a liveborn with a chromosome abnormality of any kind. The risk for older women is higher. CVS and subsequent chromosome study will detect these birth defects. Cleft palate is not detectable by analysis of CVS. CF and thalassaemia are both automsomal recessive disorders. For specific DNA diagnosis including prenatal diagnosis, both mutations present in the proband need to be known. Death of the proband does not exclude direct DNA diagnosis if the underlying mutations can be found in both parents. Prenatal diagnosis by linkage can be used but the family study is best completed prior to the pregnancy and is not possible if material is not available from the proband. Thalassaemia can be detected by analysis of fetal blood at 18 weeks.

3.7. Which of the following statements is/are true of autosomal dominant diseases?
A   Such diseases are not manifest in the heterozygote.
B   Variability of expression is very uncommon.
C   Probability that an individual at risk will develop signs of the disorder is influenced by the penetrance.
D   One of the parents of an affected individual must be heterozygous.
E   Gonadal mosaicism is a possible explanation when a second affected child is born to unaffected parents.

3.8. Which of the following conditions are inherited in an autosomal dominant manner?
A   Cystic fibrosis.
B   Thalassaemia major.
C   Hereditary microspherocytosis.
D   Neurofibromatosis.
E   Phenylketonuria.

3.9. In a disease such as achondroplasia, in which the inheritance is invariably autosomal dominant with complete penetrance, which of the following is/are true?
A   The risk of achondroplasia in each child of an affected person is 1 in 2.
B   When an affected child is born to normal parents the risk in a subsequent pregnancy is 1 in 2.
C   There is an increased frequency of consanguinity in the parents of affected people.
D   The risk to the child of two achondroplastic parents is 100%.
E   If an unaffected child is born to an affected parent, this child is not at risk of producing future affected offspring.

3.7. C E
Autosomal dominant diseases are manifest in the heterozygote (dominant) and are the result of a gene located on a chromosome other than one of the sex chromosomes (autosomal). Many autosomal dominant diseases are characterized by extreme variability of expression, and mild and severely affected people are seen even within the same family. Penetrance is the likelihood that an individual who is heterozygous for an autosomal dominant condition will be affected (manifest the phenotype). Where penetrance is less than 100% generations may be 'skipped'. Spontaneous mutations are relatively common as a cause of autosomal dominant disorders and are the usual explanation when unaffected parents produce an affected child. Gonadal mosaicism is an alternative explanation and refers to the concept of a disease-causing mutation being present in a proportion or all of the cells of a gonad (ovary or testis). This mutation may not be present in other tissues.

3.8. C D
Hereditary microspherocytosis and neurofibromatosis are autosomal dominant diseases. Cystic fibrosis, thalassaemia major and phenylketonuria are inherited recessively.

3.9. A E
Achondroplasia is autosomal dominant (80% of cases represent new mutations). The risk to the offspring of an affected person will be 1 in 2 for each pregnancy. Consanguinity does not increase the risk in offspring unless both parents are affected. If both parents have achondroplasia, there is a 1 in 4 chance that an offspring will be *unaffected*. Complete penetrance implies that those who do not show the phenotype do not carry the mutation and therefore cannot pass it on. The gene responsible for the disorder has recently been identified as the fibroblast growth factor receptor-3 (FGFR-3), with almost all affected individuals carrying the same mutation. Prenatal diagnosis is now possible by DNA analysis.

3.10. A young couple have learnt that the wife's father, aged 42 years, has Huntington disease (Huntington chorea). They have a son and a daughter. Which of the following statements is/are true?

A   On the above information alone, each of their children has 1 chance in 4 of being affected.

B   If the wife is still unaffected by the age of 50 years, her offspring will no longer be at risk.

C   The mutation underlying this disease has not been identified.

D   Presymptomatic and prenatal diagnosis are available for all individuals at risk.

E   Huntington disease is caused by a new mutation in a high proportion of cases.

3.11. A child with tuberous sclerosis has frequent seizures and mental retardation. This condition is autosomal dominant with close to 100% penetrance and extreme variability of expression. Neither parent has either seizures or intellectual deficit. Which of the following is/are correct?

A   If a subsequent child is also affected it could be predicted to be similarly affected to the first.

B   It would be important to examine carefully and investigate the parents before advising them about recurrence risk.

C   If neither parent is affected then the recurrence risk is low.

D   Variability of expression implies that an affected individual has <1 in 2 risk of passing the mutation on to each offspring.

E   Gonadal mosaicism could explain a recurrence where neither parent is affected.

3.12. Which of the following statements is/are true of autosomal recessive conditions?

A   The great majority of affected persons are the offspring of parents who are normal to all outward appearances.

B   The rarer the abnormality, the more frequently marriages between blood relatives are found amongst the parents of affected offspring.

C   After the birth of one affected offspring, the risk for subsequent pregnancies is 1 in 4.

D   Affected persons married to homozygous normal individuals have an equal chance of producing either normal or affected offspring.

E   Provided that both individuals carry mutations within the same gene, affected persons who marry other affected persons will have affected offspring only.

45

3.10. A D

Huntington disease (HD) is an autosomal dominant condition and therefore any individual who carries the HD mutation has a 1 in 2 risk of passing it on to a child of either sex. The grandchildren of affected individuals are then at a 1 in 4 risk of carrying this faulty gene. This disease is generally a disorder of adult onset, though it can manifest at any age. It is usually not seen until 40 years of age or later. At 50 years there would still be a significant risk that the individual at risk is carrying the mutation but has not yet developed signs of the condition. The underlying mutation associated with the Huntington gene on 4p is now understood to be an unstable triplet repeat expansion (like that causing fragile X syndrome and myotonic dystrophy). Like other triplet repeat disorders, new mutations are very uncommon.

3.11 B C E

If a condition is fully penetrant then all heterozygous individuals will be affected. If a condition is described as having variability of expression this implies that there is a spectrum of severity of phenotype seen in affected individuals. One of the 'normal' parents could be mildly affected, so careful examination to look for minor features would be required. The risk to the offspring of heterozygotes is the same whether the parent is severely or mildly affected because it relates only to whether or not they carry the mutant gene. The risk is 1 in 2. Gonadal mosaicism refers to a situation where one parent is carrying the disease-causing mutation in all or part of an ovary or testis. This can explain recurrence of an autosomal dominant disorder where neither parent is affected.

3.12. A B C E

By definition autosomal recessive disorders are not manifest in the heterozygote. Generally, autosomal recessive conditions affect only members of the one sibship and affected individuals are not usually seen in earlier or subsequent generations. Consanguinity is more commonly seen amongst the parents of the very rare autosomal recessive disorders, where meeting a carrier by 'chance' is less likely. If both parents are heterozygous the risk is 1 in 4 for each offspring. Affected persons married to homozygous normal individuals will produce carrier individuals only and none of their offspring will be affected. Homozygous affected individuals produce only affected offspring unless the abnormality is due to mutations within different genes.

3.13. The incidence of a particular autosomal recessive disease is 1 in 2500. Which of the following statements is/are correct?

A The frequency of the homozygous state for the abnormal allele is 1 in 250.
B The frequency of the heterozygote state is 1 in 25.
C The chance of two carriers of this condition producing an affected child is 1 in 2 with each pregnancy.
D The gene frequency for the abnormal allele is 1 in 50.
E Unaffected siblings of an affected individual have a 2 in 3 chance of being carriers.

3.14. Which of the following is/are inherited as an autosomal recessive condition?

A Phenylketonuria.
B Cystic fibrosis.
C Factor VIII deficiency (haemophilia A).
D Neurofibromatosis.
E Congenital adrenal hyperplasia.

3.15. Jason has cystic fibrosis (CF). His parents are healthy and have two previous children. DNA testing shows that he is homozygous for the Delta F508 mutation and that his older married sister is heterozygous for the Delta F508 mutation. His brother has not had mutation analysis but his sweat test is normal. Which of the following statements is/are true?

A His sister could also have CF.
B Jason's brother has a 1 in 2 chance of being a carrier of CF.
C If the sister's husband is Chinese that couple's offspring would be at < 1% risk of CF.
D Jason is unlikely to father any offspring.
E These results are suggestive of consanguinity between Jason's parents.

3.13. B D E

The Hardy–Weinberg equilibrium describes the relationship between the normal (wild) and the abnormal (mutant) allele in the population. If p is the frequency of the normal allele and q is the frequency of the abnormal allele, then $p + q = 1$. Therefore $p^2 + 2pq + q^2 = 1$, where p^2 is equal to the frequency of the homozygous normal state, $2pq$ is the frequency of the heterozygous (carrier) state and q^2 is the frequency of the disease in the population (homozygous affected). In the example given, the frequency of the homozygous affected state (q^2) is 1/2500, so $q = 1/50$. p^2 is close to 1 so the frequency of the heterozygous state is $2pq$, i.e. 1 in 25. The gene frequency is 1 in 50. If a sibling of an affected child is known to be unaffected there are 2 chances out of 3 of that individual being a carrier (affected individuals have been eliminated).

3.14. A B E

Phenylketonuria, cystic fibrosis and congenital adrenal hyperplasia are autosomal recessive diseases. Factor VIII deficiency is X-linked recessive. Neurofibromatosis is autosomal dominant.

3.15. C D

The sister is heterozygous meaning that she has only one copy of the CF mutation (Delta F508). Both her parents carry Delta F508 so neither of them could pass on a *different* CF mutation or they would be CF affected themselves. She is, therefore, a CF carrier – not CF affected. Siblings of CF individuals, provided they do not have CF, each have a 2 in 3 chance of carrier status. Chinese are far less likely to be CF carriers than are Caucasians, in whom 1 in 25 individuals is a carrier. Therefore the risk to offspring for this couple is very low (1% is the risk if the husband is of North European/Caucasian origin.) CF males are infertile. The majority of CF individuals are homozygous for DeltaF 508. Consanguinity is unlikely in a recessive disorder where the gene frequency is relatively common.

3.16. Amanda and Alan are first cousins seeking genetic advice. They are in good health. There is no family history of inherited disorders. Which of the following statements is/are true?

A   The average incidence of birth defects in their offspring is closer to 1 in 20 than to 1 in 4.

B   The risk for birth defects in their offspring would be greater if one of their parents was the result of a first cousin marriage.

C   Their offspring are at increased risk for autosomal dominant disorders.

D   Their offspring are at increased risk for autosomal recessive disorders.

E   Their sons are at increased risk for sex-linked recessive disorders.

3.17. A 38-year-old woman has an only son in whom red/green colour blindness is diagnosed. Her brother is also affected. Which of the following statements is/are correct?

A   The condition is X-linked dominant.

B   Any future daughters will be carriers.

C   All of the son's daughters will be a carriers.

D   Her son has a 1 in 2 risk of producing affected male offspring.

E   All sons of affected females will be affected.

3.18. Bertha has a brother and a maternal uncle with haemophilia A. Her sister has a mild but significant bleeding tendency. Which of the following statements is/are true?

A   The risk of haemophilia in Bertha's first offspring, if male, is 1 in 4.

B   The bleeding tendency in Bertha's sister indicates that the defective gene is autosomal in this family.

C   Bertha's mother is an obligate carrier.

D   Prenatal diagnosis of haemophilia A is possible.

E   If Bertha has three unaffected sons, this would influence the probability that she is a carrier.

3.16. A D
First cousins are more likely than unrelated individuals to be carrying the same faulty recessive genes. Therefore their children are at greater risk of being affected by autosomal recessive disorders. The risk of autosomal dominant disorders and sex-linked recessive disorders is not increased though there may be some increase in the risk for multifactorial conditions. If one of the normal parents is themselves the product of a first cousin marriage, this does not increase their risk.

3.17. C E
Red/green colour blindness is an X-linked recessive disease. There is a 1 in 2 chance that any daughter of a carrier will also be a carrier. All daughters of an affected son will be carriers but affected males never have affected sons. Sons of affected females are always affected.

3.18. A C D E
Haemophilia is an X-linked recessive disorder. The chance that Bertha is a carrier is 1 in 2 and therefore the chances of having a child with haemophilia is 1 in 8. If the child is male the risk is 1 in 4. The family tree is consistent with X-linked inheritance. The fact that Bertha's mother has produced an affected boy and that she has an affected brother means that she must be a carrier. Some carrier females show a mild bleeding tendency. Prenatal diagnosis of haemophilia A can be achieved by direct mutation analysis in families where the mutation is known and is frequently possible in other families by indirect DNA methods (family linkage study). Factor VIII levels can also be assayed in fetal blood. For a possible carrier, the birth of each unaffected son decreases the likelihood that she is a carrier (Bayes' theorem).

3.19. Julie's son Noel is 2 and a half years old and has delayed motor milestones. Recently he has begun to stumble and rises from the floor by pushing up on his knees with his hands. His calves look well developed and his creatine kinase (CK) is 4000 u/l. Julie's brother died of muscular dystrophy aged 23 years. Her sister is planning a pregnancy. A deletion within the dystrophin gene is demonstrated in DNA from Noel's blood. Which of the following statements regarding Noel's condition is/are true?

A Julie's carrier status remains in doubt.

B Based on the information above, Julie's sister is at 1 in 2 risk of carrier status.

C If Julie's sister is shown to have a normal CK result then she is not a carrier.

D Prenatal diagnosis is possible for Julie but not her sister.

E If Julie's sister already has three unaffected sons this fact could be used to modify her risk

3.20. An 18-year-old girl has a full brother and two maternal half brothers who are mentally retarded. The youngest affected half-brother, born when his mother was 39, has Down syndrome (karyotype 47 XY + 21). Both the other retarded males are normal in physical appearance and chromosomal analysis (including special culture for fragile X) shows normal results. Concerning the risk of mental retardation in this girl's offspring, which of the following is/are true?

A It is likely that her mother is a carrier of fragile X mental retardation.

B The girl in question has a 1 in 2 risk of being a carrier for X-linked retardation.

C The risk of her offspring having trisomy 21 is greater than 1%.

D Prenatal diagnosis is possible by chromosome analysis of cells obtained by amniocentesis.

E She has a 1 in 8 risk of bearing retarded offspring.

3.21. In genetic terms, 'anticipation'

A implies increasing severity of the disease in subsequent generations.

B is associated with expansion of triplet repeats in the DNA sequence.

C is seen in Huntington disease.

D indicates that the disease will manifest later.

E is a spurious observation due to selection bias.

3.19. B E

The condition is Duchenne muscular dystrophy which is X-linked recessive in its inheritance. Julie is an obligate carrier by pedigree analysis alone. Julie's sister has an *a priori* carrier risk of 1 in 2, but with each unaffected son she produces it becomes less and less likely that she is a carrier. A repeatedly elevated CK will confirm carrier status but a normal CK does not eliminate carrier status as many carriers have normal CK levels. Once the underlying mutation is known, prenatal diagnosis can be offered to all possible carriers in the family.

3.20. B E

The pedigree is strongly suggestive of non-specific X-linked mental retardation. Specific cytogenetic studies have ruled out fragile X mental retardation as the underlying cause of the problem in these brothers. The risk to this girl's offspring is not increased by the fact that her mother gave birth to a child with non-disjunction trisomy 21. Pedigree information suggests the mother is a carrier of non-specific X-linked mental retardation. This then infers a 1 in 2 risk that her daughter is a carrier, which in turn implies a 1 in 8 risk to her offspring. If the affected retarded males have not shown karyotypic abnormalities (including fragile X), an analysis of the chromosomes of the pregnancy will not be useful in providing prenatal diagnosis.

3.21. A B C

Anticipation is a genetic term which implies that the phenotype (clinical features) of a disease becomes progressively more severe and/or manifests at an earlier age in subsequent generations. It is associated with expansion of a trinucleotide repeat in the genomic DNA sequence of that gene. Diseases showing this feature include fragile X mental retardation, myotonic dystrophy, Huntington disease and several forms of spinocerebellar atrophy. The original observations of anticipation were incorrectly thought to represent spurious selection bias.

3.22. In multifactorial inheritance, factors affecting the risk to relatives are
A   the presence of multiple affected family members
B   the age of the parent at the time of proband's birth.
C   closeness of the relationship to the proband.
D   the presence of severe and/or early onset disease in the proband.
E   whether or not the proband is shown to have a normal karyotype.

3.23. Which of the following conditions is determined by polygenic inheritance?
A   Galactosaemia.
B   Talipes.
C   Meningomyelocoele.
D   Polydactyly.
E   Turner syndrome.

3.24. A 20-year-old woman in her first pregnancy has a routine 18-week ultrasound and lumbosacral spina bifida is diagnosed. After the pregnancy is terminated she is concerned about the risk for recurrence in a subsequent pregnancy. Which of the following statement(s) is/are true?
A   The risk would be greater if she was over 35.
B   The risk depends on whether the next child is female or male.
C   The risk can be lowered by about 70% by administrating folic acid prior to and during pregnancy.
D   A high resolution ultrasound scan at 18 weeks will detect only about 20% of recurrences.
E   The risk of anencephaly is less than 1 in 1000.

3.25. Which of the following statements is/are true of chromosome abnormalities?
A   The chromosome number (chromosomes per cell) is the same with a balanced reciprocal translocation as with a balanced Robertsonian translocation.
B   Recurrent spontaneous abortion is a valid indication for chromosome studies.
C   If a baby has Down syndrome due to a 21/14 translocation, one or the other parent must be a balanced translocation carrier.
D   The extra chromosome in non-disjunction trisomy 21 is more often of maternal than of paternal origin.
E   Trisomy 21 is the most frequent single anomaly associated with first trimester spontaneous abortion.

3.22. A C D
The risk to relatives is influenced by the closeness of the relationship to the proband, the degree of heritability of the disorder, whether the proband is of the more commonly affected sex, whether he or she has severe or early onset disease and whether or not there are multiple family members affected.

3.23. B C
Neural tube defects such as meningomyelocoele are inherited in a multifactorial manner. Talipes is associated with a recurrence risk of about 3% after the birth of an affected child, which suggests multifactorial causes. Some cases of talipes are due to abnormal posture *in utero*. All forms of galactosaemia are autosomal recessive in inheritance. Polydactyly not associated with any other abnormality is autosomal dominant with incomplete penetrance. Turner syndrome is due to a chromosome abnormality involving loss (45,X) or rearrangement of the X chromosome.

3.24. C
For a couple in whom a neural tube defect occurred in the first fetus the risk of recurrence may be as high as 4–5% (risk for high-risk populations). This risk applies to all types of neural tube defect: spina bifida, encephalocoele and anencephaly. Folic acid 5 mg daily for one month prior to conception and for 3 months after will reduce this risk by about 70%. High-resolution ultrasound scanning at 18 weeks by an experienced operator can detect almost all neural tube defects. Risk is independent of sex.

3.25. B D
In individuals with a balanced Robertsonian translocation the chromosome number is 45 instead of the usual 46. In balanced reciprocal translocations chromosome number is 46. Six percent of couples who have had more than three miscarriages will be found to be carriers of a balanced chromosome rearrangements such as translocations; this is the underlying reason for pregnancy loss. Among families of infants with translocation Down syndrome, neither parent is shown to be a carrier approximately 50% of the time. The extra copy of chromosome 21 in non-disjunction trisomy 21 is more frequently of maternal than paternal origin, and the most frequent sex chromosome anomaly associated with early spontaneous abortion is 45,X (Turner syndrome).

3.26. Which of the following statements is/are true of Down syndrome?

A   If the parents are in their early twenties the karyotype is likely to show translocation Down syndrome.

B   In more than 90% of cases, parents' chromosomes are normal.

C   If the karyotype shows mosaic Down syndrome (50% 46 XX + 50% 47 XX + 21) then the phenotype will be much less severe.

D   Mortality rate *in utero* exceeds 25%.

E   The incidence among infants born to women aged 40 is more than twice that at a maternal age of 35.

3.27. Which of the following statements is/are true of individuals with Turner syndrome?

A   They frequently present with ambiguous genitalia.

B   At least 20% are fertile.

C   There is an increased incidence of systemic hypertension.

D   Puffy feet and hands can persist for longer than the first year.

E   50% show a moderate degree of intellectual retardation.

3.28. Individuals with which of the following karyotypes would generally pass for normal in society?

A   Translocation reported as 45,XX rob (13;14).

B   Trisomy 13.

C   Turner syndrome 45,X.

D   Klinefelter syndrome 47,XXY.

E   47,XYY.

3.26. B D E
Down syndrome is almost always due to simple non-disjunction trisomy 21 (95%). Most remaining cases are due to Robertsonian translocations involving chromosome 21, and the rest are mosaic in karyotype. More than 50% of trisomy 21 fetuses are spontaneously aborted during pregnancy. The overall incidence at birth is 1 in 600–800 live births. If the mother is aged 40 years the risk is about 1%, which is almost 4 times the risk at 35 years. If the infant has a translocation then the parental karyotype will be important in counselling the parents and other family members. The severity of the phenotype in Down syndrome does not depend on the karyotype.

3.27. C D
Girls with Turner syndrome are phenotypically female. Infertility is almost invariable and is due to gonadal dysgenesis. Apart from shortness, most Turner syndrome girls would pass for normal in society. About 15% have coarctation of the aorta which may present with hypertension; hypertension is also more common in this group in the absence of coarctation. Puffy feet and hands often persist beyond the first year. Turner syndrome girls often have difficulty with mathematical and spatial concepts but IQ is normal overall.

3.28. A C D E
The karyotype in A is a balanced Robertsonian translocation. Only 45 chromosomes are present but as the translocation chromosome contains all the functional portions of both chromosome 13 and 14, there is no loss of functional chromosomal material. Individuals with 47,XXY and 47,XYY frequently remain undiagnosed throughout life as the features are often mild. Turner syndrome girls are short but the majority pass easily as normal individuals in society. The majority of individuals with conditions C, D and E show no obvious intellectual deficit.

3.29. For which of the following situations is the appropriate risk for future abnormal offspring less than 1%?

A   A mother of a child with galactosaemia (incidence of 1 in 40 000) who has remarried to an unrelated individual.

B   A mother with a balanced reciprocal 1:21 translocation who presents with recurrent miscarriages.

C   A couple where the husband's brother died of Becker muscular dystrophy.

D   A couple where the 28-year-old wife's sibling had non-disjunction trisomy 18.

E   Offspring of a man with bilateral retinoblastoma.

3.30. Monozygotic twinning is associated with

A   a shared placental circulation.

B   an increased incidence of congenital malformations compared with dizygotic twins.

C   placenta and membranes from which diagnosis of monozyosity can be made readily.

D   a greater frequency than dizygotic twins.

E   an increased familial incidence.

3.31. Which of the following is/are true of neuromuscular disease?

A   The specific protein which is deficient in Becker type muscular dystrophy has been characterized.

B   Unlike Duchenne, Becker muscular dystrophy does not result in a shortened life expectancy.

C   If an infant is born with congenital myotonic dystrophy but neither parent has any complaint of muscular weakness, then the case is likely to be a spontaneous mutation.

D   Facio–scapulo–humeral muscular dystrophy is usually inherited as an autosomal recessive disorder.

E   Charcot–Marie–Tooth disease can be inherited in autosomal recessive or autosomal dominant manner, but X-linked forms have not been described.

3.29. A C D

In A the carrier mother can only run the risk of producing a second affected child if her new partner is also a carrier. An incidence of 1 in 40000 implies a carrier rate of 1 in 100 in the general population. Therefore the risk for future affected offspring is 1 in 400. For a mother with a balanced reciprocal translocation who has had multiple miscarriages the risk of future abnormal offspring is approximately 10%, though the precise risk is different for each specific translocation. Becker muscular dystrophy is X-linked recessive which means the husband is not a carrier, and he cannot pass on the mutation. Risk in D is much less than 1%. The risk to any offspring of a parent affected with bilateral retinoblastoma is about 40%.

3.30. A B

The vascular anastomosis in monozygotic twins may be artery to artery, vein to vein, or artery to vein. Monozygotic twins show a higher incidence of congenital malformations than dizygotic twins. It is not possible to establish monozygosity with 100% certainty by examination of the placenta and membranes. However, the diagnosis of dizygosity can be made with more certainty if the presence of two chorions is shown or, more reliably, the twins are of opposite sex. DNA 'fingerprinting' is now the method of choice if zygosity needs to be determined with certainty. The incidence of monozygotic twins is less than that of dizygotic twins. Monozygous twins are rarely familial but there is a familial tendency for dizygous twinning.

3.31. A

The absent/deficient protein in both Duchenne and Becker dystrophies is known as dystrophin. Becker dystrophy significantly shortens life but affected individuals live longer than those with Duchenne dystrophy. Myotonic dystrophy is characterized by an extreme paucity of new mutations. Congenitally affected infants are almost always born to affected mothers, many of whom are not aware they have the disease at the time the affected infant is born. Facio–scapulo–humeral (FSH) dystrophy is an autosomal dominant disorder characterized by extreme variability of expression. Charcot–Marie–Tooth (CMT) disease can be inherited in autosomal recessive, autosomal dominant and an X-linked manner. X-linked CMT is now recognized as the second most common type after autosomal dominant types.

3.32. Stephen and Carol's first child was affected with spinal muscular atrophy (SMA) of the infantile type (Werdnig Hoffman disease). The child died aged 8 months. They request prenatal diagnosis in a second pregnancy. The SMA gene has been localized to 5q. A linkage study is undertaken utilizing a very closely linked AC repeat marker. This marker has 3 alleles referred to as A, B and C. Which of the following would result in 100% informative prenatal diagnosis? (Clue: draw up the pedigree.)

A   Father AA and mother CC and affected child AC.
B   Father AB and mother AB and affected child AA.
C   Father AC and mother AB and affected child AB.
D   Father AB and mother AB and affected child AB.
E   Father AA and mother AC and affected child AC.

3.33 Which of the following inborn errors of metabolism is X-linked in inheritance?

A   Tay Sachs disease.
B   Fabry disease.
C   Glucose-6-phosphate dehydrogenase deficiency.
D   Menkes disease.
E   Lowe syndrome.

3.34. Which of the following statements apply to the mucopolysaccharidoses?

A   The underlying abnormality lies in the lysosomal enzymes.
B   They are all autosomal recessive.
C   A bone dysplasia is associated.
D   Cataract is a feature in all.
E   Glucose aminoglycans are deficient in urine.

3.35. Which of the following is/are true of a woman with phenylketonuria?

A   The diagnosis can be made by newborn screening.
B   Dietary management is not necessary beyond the first 4 years of life.
C   Frequency of the disorder is 1 in 1000.
D   Her offspring are at risk of intellectual deficit.
E   Even with good dietary control ovarian failure is frequently seen.

3.32. B C
In A no prediction can be made (0% informative). In B affected allele is identifiable from each parent (100% informative). C is similarly 100% informative. D is partially informative – if the second pregnancy is AA or BB then a prediction can be made but an AB result is uninformative. In E an AA result is interpretable but AC is not. Informativeness is not related to accuracy of DNA diagnosis. Accuracy depends on the closeness of the linkage between the marker and mutation in question.

3.33. B C D E
Although the vast majority of inborn errors are inherited in an autosomal recessive manner, e.g. Tay Sachs disease, Fabry disease (which is due to a deficiency of alpha-galactosidase), G6PD deficiency, Menkes' disease and Lowe syndrome are X-linked. Menkes disease is due to a defective Copper transport protein and Lowe syndrome is due to deficiency of inositol phosphate phosphatase.

3.34. A C
Lysosomal storage disorders include the mucopolysaccharidoses as well as other conditions such as gangliosidoses including GM1 and 2 and others e.g. Niemann–Pick, Tay Sachs and Gaucher diseases. Glucoseaminoglycans (GAGS) are present in increased amounts in urine. The specific enzyme defect, where known, can be measured in leucocytes. Cataract is not seen in Hunter syndrome (MPSII) and is not a feature in several of the other MPS disorders, e.g. Sanfilippo and Sly syndromes.

3.35. A D
PKU is most frequently diagnosed by newborn screening, which is routinely carried out in many countries. The most common method involves analysis of blood spots collected at 3–5 days of age. The incidence is 1 in 25 000. Dietary management gives good results overall and needs to be continued at least into adolescence. In affected females treatment needs to be strictly observed prior to conception and throughout pregnancy, as the risk of mental retardation in offspring is considerable due to high phenylalanine levels in the mother. Treated females with galactosaemia (not PKU) have a risk of ovarian dysfunction.

3.36. A 15-year-old girl has myopathy, encephalopathy, lactic acidosis and stroke-like episodes. Her mother and brother have a similar illness. Which of the following statements apply to this condition?

A   It is due to a point mutation in the mitochondrial DNA.
B   It is X-linked dominant.
C   It can be diagnosed by PCR.
D   50% of the brother's children will be affected.
E   CSF lactate and pyruvate levels will be low.

3.37. Which of the following techniques is/are used for DNA testing?

A   Polymerase chain reaction.
B   Chromosome analysis.
C   Genetic probes.
D   Southern blotting.
E   *In situ* hybridization.

3.38. Polymerase chain reaction can be carried out

A   in routine laboratories without special precautions.
B   to diagnose single gene defects.
C   on old tissue samples.
D   to diagnose infections.
E   to detect a small number of cancer cells.

3.36. A C
MELAS (Mitochondrial myopathy with Encephalopathy, Lactic Acidosis and Stroke-like episodes) is a disorder of mitochondrial DNA due to a point mutation which is maternally inherited, as the mitochondria of the zygote are derived from the ovum. Typically, all children of mothers carrying mitochondrial mutation in their ova will inherit that mutation, although the clinical consequences are very variable within families. Children of affected men do not inherit the disease since they do not receive any mitochondria from the father's sperm. The CSF lactic and pyruvate levels are high or normal.

3.37. A C D E
PCR allows amplification of a specific DNA sequence which can then be further analysed. It can be used to analyse small or impure samples. Genetic probes are nucleic acid bases arranged in a sequence which allow detection of whether genomic sequence is present, deleted or altered. In Southern blotting the DNA sample is cut into fragments at specific sites by enzymes. The fragments are size sorted by electrophoresis and analysed by radiolabelled gene probes. *In situ* hybridization is used to detect deletions and rearrangements of chromosomal DNA. Chromosomal analysis is useful for gross abnormalities including large deletions or duplications/insertions of chromosomal material.

3.38. B C D E
The use of PCR requires meticulous care to prevent contamination. Separate work areas (or preferably separate laboratories), gowns and equipment should be used for pre- and post-amplification processing of samples. PCR has been applied extensively for diagnosis of single gene defects either directly, by detection of mutations, or indirectly by linkage analysis. Dried blood, hair roots, paraffin-fixed slides and even extremely old tissue can be used as DNA is resistant to degradation. It is particularly useful for diagnosis of infections caused by slowly growing organisms such as mycobacteria, which are difficult to culture. It has been used to detect cancer cells persisting after treatment in the management of malignant disease.

4 Fetal and neonatal medicine

4.1. Which of the following statements is/are correct about fetal growth and development?

A   Respiratory movements do not occur until birth.
B   Swallowing movements commence as early as 14 weeks gestation.
C   Haemoglobin is primarily HbF.
D   Organogenesis occurs in the second trimester. ✗ 1st trimester
E   The third trimester is one of growth rather than differentiation.

4.2. Routine newborn screening on a filter paper blood spot is possible for which of the following conditions?

A   Thalassaemia major.
B   Hypothyroidism.
C   G-6-PD deficiency.
D   Cystic fibrosis.
E   Galactosaemia. → check

4.3 Which of the following statements is/are true of a normal full-term infant on the first day of life?

A   Fluid requirements are 100 ml/kg on the first day. ✗ 60
B   The average head circumference is 29 cm. ✗ 35
C   The urinary output is 1–3 ml/kg. ✓
D   A true blood glucose of 2 mmol/l is within the normal range. ✓
E   The average blood pressure is 50–60 mmHg. ✓

4.4. In a full-term infant weighing 3.5 kg

A   the digestive tract lacks some of the enzymes needed for digestion of milk products.
B   supplemental iron therapy is indicated from the age of 3 weeks.
C   subconjuctival haemorrhage is most likely to be due to strangulation by cord around the neck. → any cause that ↑ venous return to head.
D   vaginal bleeding indicates haemorrhagic disease.
E   blood volume is about 300 ml.

4.1. B C E
Fetal respiratory movements can be seen by ultrasound as early as 18 weeks' gestation. Swallowing movements are seen by the 14th week. The haemoglobin of the fetus is mainly HbF which carries more oxygen than adult haemoglobin (HbA). Organogenesis occurs in the first trimester (mainly the first 8 weeks of pregnancy). In the third trimester there is maturation of body functions and gain in weight.

4.2. B C D E
Screening for hypothyroidism, cystic fibrosis, G-6-PD deficiency and galactosaemia can be carried out on blood (spot) collected on filter paper.

4.3. C D E
The fluid requirements of a full-term infant on the first day of life are 60 ml/kg, the average head circumference is 35 cm and urinary output is 1–3 ml/kg. The reported blood sugar range is 1.5–4 mmol/l. The average blood pressure is 50–60 mmHg.

4.4. E
A full-term infant has all the enzymes necessary for digestion of milk. Iron therapy is not needed as the infant has adequate stores of iron derived from the mother. Subconjuctival haemorrhage usually occurs because of obstruction of venous return from the head and is not necessarily due to strangulation by cord around the neck. Spurious menstruation occurs in female newborn infants due to withdrawal of maternal and placental oestrogens. Blood volume is about 8–10% of body weight.

4.5. Which of the following statements concerning newborn babies is/are correct?

A Jaundice occurring on the first day of life is pathological.

B Hydrocoele should be drained as early as possible to avoid testicular atrophy. *⇒ most resolve spontaneously*

C Eosinophilic rash (erythema toxicum) is an allergic manifestation.

D Ductus arteriousus usually closes physiologically within 48 h. *(due to ↑O₂*

E Facial petechiae at birth are indicative of haemorrhagic disease. *tension in aorta)*

4.6. Which of the following statements is/are correct?

A Gestational age of 35 weeks + 6 days should be considered as 36 weeks.

B Preterm is defined as a gestation of less than 35 weeks.

C Small-for-date babies are more common than large-for-date babies. *(same)*

D Postmature infants are more than 42 weeks' gestation.

E Neonatal period extends up to 30 days of life. *✗ 28 days of life*

4.7. Which of the following definitions is/are correct?

A Stillbirth: death *in utero* prior to the complete expulsion of products of conception.

B Neonatal death: death of a live-born infant in the first 28 days.

C Premature infant: an infant weighing 2.5 kg or less at birth.

D Perinatal death: includes both death *in utero* after 20 weeks' gestation (or birth weight 400 g or more) and death after delivery in the first 28 days of life.

E Neonatal mortality rate: neonatal deaths divided by 1000 total births.

4.8. In which of the following conditions is polyhydramnios a recognized complication of pregnancy?

A Anencephaly.

B Oesophageal atresia.

C Maternal diabetes mellitus.

D Renal agenesis. *⇒ oligohydramnios*

E Ileal atresia.

4.9. Which of the following statements is/are true of alpha-fetoprotein (AFP)?

A Its concentration in amniotic fluid is increased in fetal intestinal atresia.

B In amniotic fluid its concentration is maximum at 12–14 weeks' gestation. *✗ 14–15*

C In maternal serum its maximum concentration is at 26 weeks' gestation.

D The main site of synthesis of AFP is the fetal spinal cord.

E AFP levels are normal in closed meningocoeles.

↑ is open ✓ + answer

65

4.5. A D

Jaundice appearing on the first day of life is usually haemolytic or due to intrauterine infection. Most hydrocoeles in the neonatal period resolve spontaneously. The aetiology of eosinophilic rash is not known. Physiological closure of the ductus arteriosus occurs within few hours of birth due to high oxygen tension in the aorta. Facial petechiae can occur in any condition which causes obstruction of flow of blood from the head and neck.

4.6. D

Gestational age is stated as completed weeks. A preterm infant is defined as an infant less than 37 weeks' gestation (i.e. 36 weeks, 6 days). Neonatal period is defined as the first 28 days of life. Infants who are small-for-dates (less than 10th percentile) and large-for-dates (more than 90th percentile) are equal in number. Postmaturity is more than 42 weeks' gestation.

4.7. B D

Stillbirth is death of a fetus of more than 20 weeks' gestation prior to complete expulsion (or delivery) or if gestational age is unknown, fetal weight is 400 g or more. Neonatal death is death of a live-born infant in the first 28 days of life. Prematurity is gestational age of less than 37 weeks. Perinatal deaths include both stillbirths and neonatal deaths. Neonatal mortality rate is neonatal deaths per 1000 live births.

4.8. A B C

Polyhydramnios may occur in association with any major congenital malformation, but particularly with anencephaly. It has a recognized association with maternal diabetes. Oesophageal atresia causes polyhydramnios because the fetus is unable to swallow the amniotic fluid. In renal agenesis there is oligohydramnios. Midgut and colonic atresias do not affect the volume of liquor amnii.

4.9. A E

Alpha-fetoprotein level in the amniotic fluid is a maximum at 14–18 weeks of gestation. Maternal serum concentrations are highest at 16–18 weeks of gestation. It is synthesized by the fetal liver. Levels are raised in anencephaly and open meningomyelocoeles but not in closed meningocoeles. Its concentration in amniotic fluid is also increased by the presence of fetal blood, fetal abortion or death, Rh disease, congenital nephrosis, omphalocoele, intestinal atresia and Meckel's syndrome.

4.10. Which of the following statements is/are true of second trimester prenatal diagnosis?

A   Diagnosis of neural tube defect requires cultivation of amniocytes.
B   It is possible to diagnose polycystic disease of kidneys.
C   The risk of fetal death (i.e. unintended abortion) associated with amnio-centesis is about 5% in experienced hands.
D   DNA for diagnostic testing may be obtained from amniotic fluid.
E   Examination of maternal blood may lead to diagnosis of neural tube defect.

4.11. Central nervous system abnormalities associated with the fetal alcohol syndrome include

A   mild to moderate mental retardation.
B   microcephaly.
C   irritability in the neonatal period.
D   hyperactivity in childhood.
E   macroscopic changes in the brain.

4.12. A 2.1 kg full-term infant becomes irritable and develops coarse tremors at 36 h of age. He feeds poorly and has diarrhoea and nasal stuffiness. Which of the following statements is/are true?

A   The most likely diagnosis is hypoglycaemia.
B   The most appropriate treatment for this infant is 10% calcium gluconate.
C   The patient should be isolated.
D   The mother should be tested for hepatitis B antigen.
E   The infant is at risk of developing hyperpyrexia.

4.13. Which of the following statements is/are true in newborn infants?

A   The most useful indicator of response to resuscitation is heart rate.
B   A low 1-min Apgar score correlates well with long-term prognosis.
C   Hypoxia is more likely to cause brain damage in preterm babies than in full-term babies.
D   A normal cord blood IgM excludes a congenital viral infection.
E   Convulsions following hypoxia in full-term infants indicate a poor prognosis.

4.10. B D E

Diagnosis of neural tube defect is made by measurement of alpha-fetoprotein in amniotic fluid or maternal serum and by ultrasound. The size of the kidneys can be clearly defined during the second trimester of pregnancy. The risk of abortion following amniocentesis is about 1%. DNA may be obtained from the amniotic cells in the amniotic fluid for diagnosis.

4.11. A B C D E

Alcohol causes alterations in growth and morphogenesis which will result in mental retardation, microcephaly, irritability in the neonatal period, hyperactivity in childhood and macroscopic changes in the brain.

4.12. D E

The most likely cause of neurological symptoms (irritability, tremors), diarrhoea and nasal stuffiness is drug withdrawal, which can also present as hyperpyrexia. These infants do not require isolation. Drug addicts need to be tested for hepatitis and AIDS because of their practice of sharing needles.

4.13. A E

Heart rate rises in severely asphyxiated infants following resuscitation before sustained spontaneous respiration is established. The 1-min Apgar score does not correlate well with long-term prognosis. A better indicator of long-term prognosis is the 5-min Apgar score. Brain damage occurs more readily in the mature brain. While raised cord blood IgM occurs in congenital viral infections, it is not always present. Convulsions following hypoxia are usually due to hypoxic ischaemic encephalopathy and indicate a poor prognosis.

4.14. A 1 kg baby whose mother was given pethidine just before delivery is presented to you in the delivery room for resuscitation. He is cyanosed. His heart rate is 40/min and he is limp and apnoeic. Which of the following is/are appropriate?

A Intravenous atropine.
B Intracardiac adrenaline.
C Intravenous bolus of molar sodium bicarbonate.
D Intravenous nalorphine should be the first procedure. ⇒ only if breathing not controlled by IPPV
E External cardiac massage.

4.15. Perinatal asphyxia has been implicated in the aetiology of

A necrotizing enterocolitis.
B meconium inhalation.
C hypoglycaemia. ⇒ anaerobic metabolism of glucose
D renal failure.
E intraventricular haemorrhage.

4.16. A newborn has an asymmetrical Moro reflex. The grasp reflex is preserved for the affected arm, which is weak. There is limitation in abduction and external rotation movements of the shoulder and supination of the forearm. The neurological lesion involves

A motor cortex on contralateral side.
B third and fourth cervical nerves.
C fifth and sixth cervical nerves.
D seventh and eighth cervical nerves.
E first and second thoracic nerves.

4.17. Which of the following statements is/are correct for the newborn?

A More than 90% of surfactant phosphotidylcholine (PC) is recycled.
B There is very little catabolism of exogenously adminstered PC.
C Exogenously administered PC is recycled like endogenously produced PC.
D Surfactant protein A is essential for surfactant biophysical properties.
E Surfactant proteins B and C enhance the spread of phospholipids at the air–liquid interface of alveoli.

69

4.14. E
The principles of resuscitation are A (clear Airways), B (Breathing) and C (Circulation). In this infant after clearing the airways, the infant should be given intermittent positive pressure respiration (IPPR) together with external cardiac massage. The administration of drugs is inappropriate prior to ABC. If the circulation fails to imrpove, it is more appropriate to administer a plasma expander rather than sodium bicarbonate, atropine or intracardiac adrenaline. There is no urgency to give nalorphine as the breathing can be controlled by IPPR.

4.15. A B C D E
Perinatal asphyxia causes necrotizing enterocolitis as a result of ischaemia of gut, passage of meconium into the liquor leading to inhalation, hypoglycaemia due to anaerobic metabolism of glycogen, renal failure due to renal tubular necrosis and intraventricular haemorrhage due to cerebral ischaemia and disturbances of cerebral blood flow.

4.16. C
The muscles innervated by the fifth and sixth cervical roots are deltoid, biceps, brachioradialis and supinator, which control some of the affected movements described in the stem.

4.17. A B C E
The recycling of surfactant is more efficient in the newborn than the adult (90% or more compared with 50%). Forty percent of exogenously administered PC can be recovered by alveolar lavage and the remainder from lung tissue. It is taken up by type II pneumocytes and recycled. The functions of surfactant protein A are to prevent inhibition of surfactant by serum proteins and regulation of secretion and re-uptake of dipalmitoyl PC by type II pneumocytes, and that of surfactant proteins B and C are lipid adsorption and spread of phospholipid at the air–liquid interface.

4.18. A full-term infant weighing 2.4 kg develops tachypnoea, grunting and intercostal recession. Full blood count shows haematocrit 75, WBC 25 000/ml (60% neutrophils, 30% lymphocytes, 8% monocytes, 2% bands). Which of the following statements is/are correct?

A   Chest X-ray is likely to show a reticulogranular (snow storm) appearance.
B   The white cell count supports a diagnosis of sepsis.
C   The infant is dehydrated.
D   The high haematocrit is the possible cause of the respiratory distress.
E   The infant is at risk of developing pulmonary haemorrhage.

4.19. An infant delivered at 32 weeks' gestation develops respiratory distress soon after birth with marked chest recession. At the age of 4 h he has a cyanotic episode. Chest X-ray shows ground-glass appearance with an air bronchogram. This presentation is consistent with the diagnosis of

A   hyaline membrane disease.
B   meconium aspiration.
C   wet lung.
D   bacterial infection.
E   tracheo-oesophageal fistula.

4.20. Which of the following conditions is/are recognized as being associated with respiratory difficulties in newborn infants?

A   Funnel chest (pectus excavatum).
B   Oesophageal atresia.
C   Oligohydramnios.
D   Bilateral choanal atresia.
E   Micrognathia (receded chin) with cleft palate.

4.18. D E
The likely diagnoses in this infant are respiratory distress due to high viscosity (as a result of high haematocrit) or infection. Chest X-ray may be normal or show evidence of congestive cardiac failure or patchy pneumonia. Infants with high haematocrit have low platelet levels and develop disseminated intravascular coagulation with a bleeding diathesis including pulmonary haemorrhage. Infants with sepsis are more likely to develop leucopenia and neutropenia than leucocytosis. An immature (band) to total white cell count ratio of more than 0.2 strongly supports a diagnosis of sepsis.

4.19. A D
Prematurity, respiratory distress syndrome and the X-ray appearances described are consistent with hyaline membrane disease, which is indistinguishable from bacterial infection. The X-ray appearances are not consistent with meconium aspiration, wet lung or tracheo-oesophageal fistula.

4.20. B C D E
Funnel chest causes no respiratory symptoms. The respiratory difficulties in oesophageal atresia are due to aspiration of secretions into the lung, in oligohydramnios are due to lung hypoplasia, in bilateral choanal atresia arise because newborn infants are obligate nose breathers, and in micrognathia with cleft palate (Pierre–Robin syndrome) are due to obstruction of breathing by falling back of the tongue.

4.21. A female infant, birth weight 1.2 kg, required intermittent positive pressure ventilation from birth. She needed 60–80% oxygen for the first 5 days and subsequently required 40–50% oxygen. She was extubated at the age of 1 month but remained oxygen-dependent for another 90 days. Which of the following statements apply to this infant?

A   In the early stages of the disease parenteral dexamethasone has been shown to improve the respiratory status.

B   Histology of the bronchi would show mucosal hyperplasia and metaplasia.

C   The chest X-ray findings may be similar to those seen in aspiration pneumonia.

D   The infant is likely to require multiple hospital admissions after discharge.

E   The infant is likely to have hyper-reactive airways.

4.22. A full-term infant weighing 3.5 kg has had respiratory distress from birth. His oxygen requirements increased progressively over the first 12 h and arterial blood gases show pH 7.26, PCO_2 30 mmHg, PO_2 35 mmHg in 100% oxygen. Echocardiogram shows no evidence of congenital heart disease other than a patent ductus arteriosus. Which of the following statements is/are correct?

A   The patient should be hyperventilated.

B   Nitric oxide has been demonstrated to be effective in the treatment of these patients.

C   The patients should be given indomethacin.

D   The patient has respiratory acidosis.

E   Treatment with extracorporeal membrane oxygenator (ECMO) can save 60–80% of such infants.

4.23. Diaphragmatic hernia in the newborn

A   is more common on the right side than the left.

B   is associated with pulmonary hypoplasia.

C   may be asymptomatic.

D   characteristically causes vomiting.

E   has more than a chance association with malrotation of the gut.

4.21. A B C D E
This infant has bronchopulmonary dysplasia (BPD). Some of these patients can be weaned off the ventilator in the early stage following a short course of parenteral steroids. Histological changes include peribronchial small muscle hypertrophy, fibrous tissue in basement membrane and mucosal hyperplasia and metaplasia. Recurrent aspiration due to gastro-oesophageal reflux is indistinguishable from bronchopulmonary dysplasia and has also been implicated in the aetiology of BPD. Infants with BPD have a family history of asthma and have hyper-reactive airways. These infants develop respiratory failure following respiratory viral infections, necessitating hospitalization.

4.22. A B E
In the presence of a low Po_2, a normal Pco_2 and a normal heart, the diagnosis is persistent pulmonary hypertension of newborn. These infants respond to treatment with hyperventilation and nitric oxide, which has been shown to be the endothelial dilating release factor. Up to 80% of these infants with an oxygen index of more than 40 survive following treatment with ECMO. Indomethacin is contraindicated. The blood gases indicate that the patient has metabolic acidosis.

4.23. B C E
Diaphragmatic hernia is more common on the left, is associated with pulmonary hypoplasia because of the gut contents in the thorax and does not cause vomiting. There is often incomplete rotation of the gut. Some patients may be diagnosed on routine chest X-ray.

4.24. A baby of 40 weeks' gestation is born weighing 2000 g. Which of the following statements is/are likely to be true of this infant?
A   He is premature.
B   He is at risk of developing hypoglycaemia.
C   His mother is a prediabetic.
D   He is at risk of developing meconium aspiration.
E   His head circumference is likely to be on a similar percentile to his weight.

4.25. A 25-year-old para 1 mother gave birth to twin boys at 38 weeks' gestation. Twin A weighed 3200 g and twin B weighed 2400 g at birth. Which of the following statements is/are correct?
A   The weight of twin B is appropriate for gestational age and twin A is large for gestational age.
B   The weight of twin A is appropriate for gestational age and twin B is small for gestational age.
C   Neither infant is appropriate weight for twins at 38 weeks' gestation.
D   Both infants are large for twins at 38 weeks' gestation.
E   There is an increased risk in twin B of hypoglycaemia.

4.26. Which of the following have more than a chance association with the small-for-dates infant?
A   A high perinatal mortality.
B   Congenital malformation.
C   Permanent physical or mental retardation.
D   Idiopathic respiratory distress syndrome (hyaline membrane disease).
E   High haematocrit.

4.27. Which of the following neonatal problems is/are seen more frequently in the infant of diabetic mothers?
A   Hypoglycaemia.
B   Hyaline membrane disease.
C   Polycythaemia.
D   Hyperbilirubinaemia.
E   Congenital malformations.

4.24. B D
This baby is a small-for-dates infant born at term and is likely to have hypogly-caemia and intrapartum asphyxia which may cause meconium aspiration. Infants of prediabetic mothers are large-for-dates. As the head continues to grow in spite of intrauterine growth retardation the head circumference is like-ly to be on a higher percentile than the weight.

4.25. B E
The average weight of twins at term is 3.3–3.5 kg. A weight of 2.4 kg is below the 10th percentile. Twin B is likely to develop hypoglycaemia because he is small-for-dates.

4.26. A B C E
Small-for-dates infants have intrauterine stress which results in increased peri-natal morbidity, mortality and high haematocrit. Permanent physical or men-tal retardation may occur if the aetiology is intrauterine infection or chromo-somal abnormality. There is a strong association between congenital malfor-mations and small-for-dates infants. Idiopathic respiratory distresss syndrome is less likely to occur because intrauterine stress results in maturation of lung.

4.27. A B C D E
Infants of diabetic mothers will develop hypoglycaemia (because of increased production of insulin by the infant's pancreas) and hyaline membrane disease, especially if the diabetes is poorly controlled. These infants have polycythaemia and are likely to develop hyperbilirubinaemia. Infants of diabetic mothers tend to have neurological malformations (hydrocephalus, spina bifida, sacral agene-sis) congenital heart disease and left microcolon.

4.28. Which of the following statements is/are true?

A   Jaundice appearing 12 h after birth would suggest a greatly impaired glucuronyl transferase activity.

B   During fetal life products of fetal haemoglobin breakdown are cleared by passage into the amniotic fluid.

C   There is no risk of kernicterus in biliary atresia.

D   Biliary atresia is readily distinguished from neonatal hepatitis by liver function testing.

E   In newborn infants, beta-thalassaemia increases risk of hyperbilirubinaemia.

4.29. Which of the following statements is/are true of physiological jaundice?

A   It rarely (<5%) presents before the age of 24 h.

B   It is due mainly to temporarily impaired hepatic clearance of bilirubin.

C   In premature infants it may persist for 3–4 weeks.

D   Direct bilirubin levels may be as high as indirect bilirubin levels.

E   It may cause kernicterus.

4.30. Which of the following conditions have more than a chance association with non-conjugated hyperbilirubinaemia in the first month of life?

A   Hypothyroidism.

B   Breast feeding.

C   Biliary atresia.

D   Beta-thalassaemia major.

E   Intestinal obstruction.

4.31. Which of the following cause conjugated hyperbilirubinaemia persisting beyond 14 days of life?

A   Breast milk jaundice.

B   Galactosaemia.

C   Congenital hypothyroidism.

D   Biliary atresia.

E   Congenital syphilis.

4.28. C
Jaundice appearing in the first 24 h is usually due to haemolysis. Most fetal haemoglobin breakdown products are cleared via the placenta. In biliary atresia there is conjugated hyperbilirubinaemia which does not cause kernicterus. The results of liver function testing (enzymes, alkaline phosphatase) may be similar in both neonatal hepatitis and biliary atresia. There is no increased risk of hyperbilirubinaemia due to beta-thalassaemia. Newborn infants normally have haemoglobin F.

4.29. A B C
Physiological jaundice rarely appears before the age of 24–48 h and is due mainly to hepatic immaturity. It persists longer in premature infants. Direct bilirubin levels are less than 10% of the total bilirubin. Levels are never high enough to cause kernicterus.

4.30. A B E
Unconjugated hyperbilirubinaemia persists in hypothyroidism due to slow metabolism. In breast-fed infants and intestinal obstruction there is an increased load of bilirubin from the enterohepatic circulation. As the haemoglobin of a normal full-term newborn infant is about 70% HbF there is no increase in bilirubin load in beta-thalassaemia major in the newborn.

4.31. B D E
The direct hyperbilirubinaemia in galactosaemia and congenital syphilis is due to destruction of liver architecture. In biliary atresia it is due to obstruction of flow of the bile. Breast milk jaundice and congenital hypothyroidism cause unconjugated hyperbilirubinaemia.

4.32. Which of the following statements is/are correct?

A A platelet count of 50 000/ml is normal in a full-term infant aged 12 h.

B There is an increase in haemoglobin level within 3 h of birth.

C The gradual fall in haemoglobin in the first 2 weeks of life is due to instability of fetal haemoglobin.

D Anaemia in a premature infant aged 4 weeks is most likely to be due to poor iron stores.

E Blood loss is the most common cause of non-haemolytic anaemia in the newborn.

4.33. A 32-year-old gravida 2, para 1, group O Rh-negative woman delivers her second child at 38 weeks' gestation. During her pregnancy her Rh antibodies titre rose from 1:8 to 1:32. The cord blood examination shows blood group A Rh-positive, Coombs' test negative, serum bilirubin 35 μmol/l. Which of the following statements is/are correct?

A The baby does not have Rh-isoimmunization.

B The mother should be given anti-D gammaglobulin within 3 days of delivery.

C The baby is at high risk of developing hyperbilirubinaemia requiring phototherapy.

D The rise in antibody titre during the pregnancy was unrelated to the baby's Rh status.

E The mother should have undergone amniocentesis during her pregnancy.

4.34. Which of the following statements is/are true of an infant born with erythroblastosis due to Rh isoimmunization?

A His mother should be given 1 ml of anti-D gammaglobulin within 72 h of delivery.

B Acidosis will increase the risk of kernicterus in the presence of hyperbilirubinaemia.

C If an exchange transfusion is required it is desirable to use blood of the mother's Rh group.

D His mother will have a positive direct Coombs' test.

E Anaemia may become increasingly a problem after the jaundice has subsided.

4.32. B E

The platelet count in a full-term infant is between 150 000 and 250 000/ml. The increase in haemoglobin level soon after birth is due to fluid moving from the vascular to the extravascular compartment. The gradual fall of haemoglobin in the first 2 weeks of life is mainly due to 'physiological hypoplasia' of marrow. Anaemia in the premature infant at 4 weeks is most likely to be due to frequent blood sampling or due to rapid growth. Blood loss (usually occurring at birth, which may be obvious, or into the maternal circulation) is the most common cause of non-haemolytic anaemia in the newborn.

4.33. A D E

A negative Coombs' test indicates there is no Rh isoimmunization. As the mother is already isoimmunized, anti-D gammaglobulin is of little use. In the absence of haemolysis, there is no cause for hyperbilirubinaemia. The rise in antibody titre during the pregnancy was non-specific and unrelated to the baby's Rh status. The only way to diagnose accurately the severity of Rh disease in the presence of rising antibody titre is by spectroscopic examination of amniotic fluid or fetal blood sampling.

4.34. B C E

In the presence of Rh isoimmunization of the mother, anti-D gammaglobulin is of no use. Acidosis increases the penetration of CSF by bilirubin and thus increases the risk of kernicterus in the presence of hyperbilirubinaemia. As the antibodies are derived from the mother, blood of the mother's Rh group is suitable for exchange transfusion since it will not be haemolysed. The mother's blood will be positive in the indirect Coombs' test. Haemolysis continues after the neonatal period for a period of 6–12 weeks (half-life of gammaglobulin is 6 weeks) and can result in anaemia.

4.35. Which of the following statements is/are true?

A   Haemorrhagic disease of the newborn is a special risk of the first few days of neonatal life.

B   Intestinal and intracranial haemorrhage are recognized complications of haemorrhagic disease.

C   Prophylactic vitamin K should be given to all newborn babies.

D   Late haemorrhagic disease may occur in infants given a single oral dose of vitamin K at birth.

E   Vitamin K_1 is contraindicated in the jaundiced newborn.

4.36. In the fetal circulation

A   there is right-to-left shunting at atrial level.

B   there is left-to-right shunting at ductal level.

C   the pulmonary artery pressure is lower than the aortic pressure.

D   oxygen saturation of the blood entering the fetal lung is lower than that of blood entering the aorta.

E   persistence of blood flow through ductus arteriosus after delivery can be abolished by prostaglandin synthetase inhibitors.

4.37. Which of the following factors predispose(s) to the maintenance of a patent ductus arteriosus in the newborn?

A   Prematurity.

B   Respiratory distress syndrome of the newborn.

C   Perinatal hypoxia.

D   High fluid intake.

E   Advanced maternal age.

4.38. A newborn infant is cyanosed. The respiratory rate is 30/min. There are no cardiac murmurs or evidence of congestive cardiac failure. When given 100% oxygen the cyanosis remains unchanged. Blood gas analysis shows PO_2 70 mmHg in air and 450 mmHg in 100% oxygen. The pH and PCO_2 are normal. Which of the following statements is/are true?

A   It is likely that the infant does not have congenital heart disease.

B   The infant will benefit from oxygen therapy.

C   The infant has normal lungs.

D   The infant should be commenced on prostaglandin to prevent closure of the ductus arteriosus.

E   The infant should be given methylene blue.

4.35. A B C D
Haemorrhagic disease is most common in the first few days of life because very little vitamin K crosses the placenta. For this reason all newborn babies need vitamin K prophylaxis. Bleeding may occur anywhere but is most serious when it occurs in the gastrointrastinal tract (blood loss) or the central nervous system (brain injury). Administration of vitamin K_1 to a jaundiced newborn is not contraindicated. However, synthetic vitamin K in large quantities causes haemolysis and can aggravate jaundice. Although late haemorrhagic disease of the newborn occurs most frequently after no vitamin K prophylaxis or after a single oral dose of vitamin K, it has been observed after intramuscular administration of vitamin K at birth.

4.36. A D E
In the fetal circulation blood by-passes the lungs by passing from the right atrium to the left atrium and from the pulmonary artery to the aorta due to high pulmonary artery pressure compared with the aortic pressures. Blood returning from the placenta is selectively directed towards the left atrium whereas that coming from the superior vena cava is directed towards the lung. Prostaglandin synthesis inhibitors such as indomethacin cause ductus arteriosus contraction and closure.

4.37. A B C D
The closure of the ductus arteriosus is caused by muscular contraction of the ductus due to high oxygen tension in the aorta. Conditions which affect these two factors will result in delayed closure. These include prematurity, respiratory distress syndrome and perinatal hypoxia. High fluid intake delays ductus closure but the mechanism is not clearly understood. Advanced maternal age does not affect ductal closure.

4.38. A C E
The blood gas analysis and the hyperoxia test indicate that the infant has methaemoglobinaemia which is treated with methylene blue.

4.39. Which of the following is/are correct regarding renal function in an infant born at 30 weeks' gestation?

A   Glomerular filtration rate, corrected for surface area, is less than in a normal adult.

B   Nephron formation can be expected to continue for at least another 6 months.

C   The ability to retain sodium is less than in a normal adult.

D   Urinary concentrating ability is equal to that of a normal adult.

E   A bladder catheter should be inserted if no urine has been passed by 24 h of age.

4.40. The incidence of hypoglycaemia in the newborn is increased in

A   large-for-date babies of diabetic mothers.

B   babies of mothers with pregnancy-induced hypertension.

C   babies which are low birth weight for gestational age.

D   polycythaemia.

E   newborn infants with haemolytic disease due to Rh incompatibility.

4.41. Neonatal hypoglycaemia

A   does not occur in infants who have been fed early.

B   causes attacks of apnoea and cyanosis.

C   does not cause mental deficiency.

D   occurs more frequently in small-for-date infants than appropriate-for-date infants.

E   may be asymptomatic.

4.42. Which of the following is/are true of neonatal urinary tract infection?

A   It is more common in twins.

B   It is commonly associated with fever and failure to thrive.

C   It may be complicated by neonatal meningitis.

D   It may be a factor contributing to neonatal jaundice.

E   It is more likely if the mother has a urinary tract infection.

with an older child or adult, renal function is poor in the newborn. ar filtration rate and the ability to concentrate sodium are not yet well developed. Nephron maturation continues for months after birth but there is no new nephron formation. Babies may pass no urine in the first 24 h of age (some of them may have passed at or before birth without it having been recorded) and therefore do not require catheterization.

4.40. A B C D E
Large-for-date infants are born to diabetic mothers who are poorly controlled and have hyperinsulinaemia which results in hypoglycaemia. Small-for-date babies are born to mothers with pregnancy-induced hypertension or intra-uterine growth retardation. These babies have poor glycogen stores and are prone to hypoglycaemia. Polycythaemia results in hypoglycaemia due to increased metabolism of the red blood cells. Infants with haemolytic disease of newborn due to Rh incompatibility develop hypoglycaemia due to hyper-insulinism, the exact mechanism of which is not known.

4.41. B D E
Early feeding will reduce the incidence of hypoglycaemia but will not prevent it in all infants. It can cause respiratory symptoms leading to cyanosis. Small-for-date infants are more likely to develop hypoglycaemia because of their low glycogen reserves and their tendency to develop perinatal asphyxia. Newborn infants with extremely low blood sugar may be asymptomatic; this has resulted in controversy about definition of hypoglycaemia. Mental deficiency is more likely to occur with symptomatic than asymptomatic hypoglycaemia.

4.42. C D E
The symptoms of neonatal urinary tract infection are non-specific. The most common presentation is septicaemia or meningitis. Jaundice may be a promi-nent symptom. Infection is often acquired *in utero*, especially if the mother has urinary tract infection. The incidence in twins is not increased.

4.43. In group B streptococcal infections in the first 5 days
A   transmission of the organism is by intrapartum exposure.
B   the treatment of choice is gentamicin.
C   virtually all infants develop meningitis.
D   the infant may appear deceptively well.
E   chest X-ray appearances are diagnostic.

4.44. Vaginal swab at 30 weeks' gestation in a 25-year-old primagravida shows group B *Streptococcus*. She is treated with ampicillin and a repeat vaginal swab shows no growth. At 38 weeks' gestation after a labour of 16 h she requires lower segment Caesarean section for cephalo-pelvic disproportion. The baby's white cell count is normal at birth. Which of the following statements is/are true?
A   The mother should have been given parenteral amoxycillin during labour.
B   If the infant is well at birth no further action is necessary.
C   If the infant has respiratory distress at birth, amoxycillin and gentamicin should be administered.
D   This infant is at risk of developing meningitis at the age of 7 days.
E   If the urine is positive for strep antigen, the infant does not definitely have colonization with group B *Streptococcus*.

4.45. A 10-day old infant develops a copious mucopurulent eye discharge. There is no periorbital cellulitis. Which of the following statements is/are true?
A   The most likely diagnosis is gonococcal ophthalmitis.
B   Routine culture of eye swab will probably show no growth.
C   The treatment of choice is topical chloroamphenicol drops or ointment.
D   The infant is at increased risk (compared with a normal infant) of developing pneumonia.
E   If untreated, the condition can persist for months.

4.46. Which of the following statements on neonatal infections is/are true?
A   Hypothermia is a recognized sign of Gram-negative septicaemia.
B   Jaundice is a recognized sign.
C   Fresh breast milk provides greater protection against neonatal infections than sterilized breast milk.
D   The incidence of neonatal infections could be reduced by having all newborn babies nursed in a single nursery.
E   Organisms normally regarded as commensals may cause serious disease in neonates.

4.43. A D
Group B streptococcal infections are transmitted during parturition and can be prevented by administration of amoxycillin during labour. The organism is most sensitive to penicillin. Meningitis usually occurs in late-onset disease. The disease is rapidly progressive, though the infant may initially appear well. Chest X-ray appearances are non-specific and can be confused with hyaline membrane disease, aspiration pneumonias and transient tachypnoea of the newborn; they may even be normal.

4.44. A C D E
As recolonization with group B streptococci can occur following successful treatment, parenteral amoxycillin or penicillin should be given during labour to prevent vertical transmission, which may be asymptomatic at birth. Ear and umbilical swabs should be obtained from the infant for culture, and close observation is required. Antibiotics should be given to symptomatic infants until the cultures resolve the diagnosis. Colonized infants are at risk of developing late-onset disease (meningitis or osteomyelitis) from 7 days to 12 weeks after birth. A negative urinary strep antigen indicates absence of colonization but a positive strep antigen may be due to passive acquired immunity (from mother).

4.45 B D E
Gonococcal ophthalmitis usually presents within the first 24 h after birth and is accompanied by periorbital cellulitis. Eye infections presenting 1 week after birth are often caused by *Chlamydia* which require special culture techniques and are resistant to chloramphenicol. The drugs of choice are sulphonamides, erythromycin or tetracyclines. The latter should not be given parenterally. These infants are at risk of developing pneumonia. The eye infection can persist for months and cause lacrimal duct stenosis.

4.46. A B C E
Neonatal infections rarely present with fever or localizing signs. Symptoms are non-specific and include hypothermia and jaundice. Fresh breast milk provides both cellular and humoral (IgA) protection against infections. Neonatal infections are usually due to cross-infection and the incidence is reduced if the nursery is small or, preferably, if the babies are nursed with their mothers. Saprophytic organisms such as *Staphyloccus epidermidis* and *Pseudomonas pyocyaneus* can cause serious infections in the newborn infant.

4.47. Herpes simplex infection in the newborn

A is usually due to type II virus.

B causes jaundice before the third day of life.

C usually requires speculum examination of the parturient mother for correct diagnosis.

D is usually acquired during delivery.

E responds promptly to intravenous cytosine arabinoside.

4.48. Congenital rubella infection has been associated with

A cataract.

B pleocytosis of the spinal fluid.

C optic nerve hypoplasia.

D diabetes mellitus.

E deafness.

4.49. In congenital rubella

A serum IgM is usually elevated at birth.

B immunoglobulins IgG and IgM decrease from birth to 3 months.

C the persistence of the infection is due to inability of the infant to produce antibodies against rubella.

D ventricular septal defect is the most common congenital heart lesion.

E the infant is not infective after the age of 1 year.

4.50. The first baby of a para 2 rubella-immune mother has congenital CMV infection. The second infant is born at term weighing 2.3 kg and with a head circumference of 29 cm. Examination of the eyes shows choroidoretinitis. Which of the following statements is/are true?

A The infant is unlikely to have congenital CMV infection.

B Congenital rubella infection cannot be excluded.

C The infant's hearing should be tested at 3-monthly intervals.

D Cord blood is likely to show raised IgM.

E The infant should be barrier nursed.

4.47. A B D
The type II virus accounts for about 75% of herpes simplex infections which are acquired during delivery (following rupture of membranes). Diagnosis in the mother is difficult and may not be obvious. Intravenous cytosine arabinoside has not been shown to be effective, though treatment with acyclovir is more encouraging. Jaundice is an early and prominent symptom.

4.48. A B D E
Congenital rubella infection causes cataract and glaucoma. Cataract is the most characteristic ocular lesion of congenital rubella but may not be recognized until after the neonatal period. CNS involvement is frequent and may present with lethargy, irritability and bulging fontanelle. Spinal fluid shows pleocytosis. The retina is involved but the optic nerve is spared. Hearing loss may also manifest later in life, which may be as late as school age. Diabetes mellitus occurs many years later due to destruction of islet cells of the pancreas

4.49. A
IgM does not cross the placenta and its presence at birth indicates a congenital infection. In congenital infections (including rubella), there is persistence of IgG because of continued infection. In congenital rubella the infection persists as the body does not recognize the rubella virus as a foreign substance and the viraemia persists for a number of years after birth. Patent ductus arteriosus is the most common congenital heart lesion.

4.50. C D
Unlike rubella, CMV infection can recur in the mother and therefore congenital CMV infection in the infant cannot be excluded. Children with congenital CMV infection can develop deafness after birth. In any congenital infection cord blood IgM is raised. CMV is endemic in most nurseries and therefore barrier nursing is not necessary.

4.51. Which of the following may produce a clinical picture in the newborn resembling severe erythroblastosis fetalis?
A Cytomegalic inclusion disease.
B *Pneumocystis carinii.*
C Congenital syphilis.
D Congenital listeriosis
E Gaucher's disease

4.52. Which of the following is/are typical of neonatal cold injury?
A Slow, shallow, irregular respiration.
B Hypoglycaemia.
C Shivering.
D Pulmonary haemorrhage.
E Pink colour.

4.53. Which of the following statements is/are true of necrotizing enterocolitis (NEC)?
A Clostridia are the primary pathogenic organisms.
B Incidence increases with decreasing gestational age.
C The pathogenesis in full-term infants is different from that in premature infants.
D The presence of gas in the portal vein is pathognomonic.
E The infant can present with intestinal obstruction a few weeks after recovering from the illness.

4.54. Which of the following statements is/are true of neonatal seizures?
A They can be exacerbated by external stimuli.
B Generalized tonic seizures without EEG changes do not respond to anticonvulsant therapy.
C Focal tonic seizures are usually associated with EEG changes.
D Myoclonic seizures are most commonly seen with metabolic disturbances.
E Seizures due to hypocalcaemia have an excellent prognosis.

4.51. A C
Erythroblastosis fetalis is associated with conditions that cause intrauterine anaemia or infection. In this question A and C are therefore correct. *Pneumocystis carinii* and congenital listeriosis are acquired during delivery or are postnatal infections. Gaucher's disease does not cause any symptoms in the newborn.

4.52. A B D E
Following cold injury an infant may look deceptively well. The skin colour is pink with a purple hue. Respirations are slow, shallow and irregular. Hypoglycaemia occurs as a result of increased metabolic needs. Most affected infants have coagulation abnormalities, including disseminated intravascular coagulation. Death is usually due to pulmonary haemorrhage. Newborn infants may be restless in a cold environment but do not exhibit shivering.

4.53. B C D E
The organisms cultured from infants with NEC are the usual prevalent gut organisms. More than 80% of reported cases of NEC occur in premature infants, the incidence increasing with decreasing gestational age. There are no consistent risk factors in premature infants. In term infants an association with birth asphyxia, polycythaemia, respiratory distress syndrome, congenital heart disease and umbilical vessel catheterization has been suggested. Gas in the gut wall and portal vein is a pathognomonic radiological sign of NEC. After recovery the infant may develop gut stricture which may present as subacute intestinal obstruction.

4.54. B C D E
Unlike jitteriness, seizures cannot be exacerbated by external stimuli or stopped by restraint. Generalized tonic seizures represent decerebrate or decorticate posturing, have no EEG changes and fail to respond to anticonvulsant therapy. Neurologists do not regard them as seizures as these postures do not conform to the strict definition of 'seizures'. Focal tonic seizures are consistently associated with EEG changes. Myoclonic seizures occur most commonly with metabolic conditions but they are also seen with structural abnormalities of the brain. Infants with hypocalcaemic seizures have no sequelae on long term follow-up.

4.55. Which of the following statements is/are true of intraventricular haemorrhage (IVH) in the newborn?

A   The pathological lesion is venous infarction.
B   The haemorrhage originates in the caudate nucleus.
C   It causes periventricular leucomalacia.
D   It can be prevented by administration of fresh frozen plasma.
E   The severity is graded by the changes observed on CT scan of the head.

4.55. A

IVH is usually asymmetrical and is caused by venous infarction due to disturbances of cerebral blood flow or cerebral venous pressure. It usually originates from the germinal matrix but sometimes from the choroid plexus (especially in mature infants). Periventricular leucomalacia is symmetrical and is due to ischaemic (arterial) white matter injury. Although premature infants have coagulation disturbances, administration of fresh frozen plasma does not prevent IVH. Grading of IVH severity is based on the findings of ultrasound of the head.

5 Infection and immunology

5.1. Blood cultures are usually positive in cases of
A   supraglottic croup (epiglottitis).
B   *Campylobacter* gastroenteritis.
C   whooping cough.
D   bronchiolitis.
E   bacterial meningitis.

5.2. Which of the following statements is/are true of *Streptococcus pyogenes* infections?
A   They account for less than 5% of upper respiratory infections in children under the age of 2 years.
B   The treatment of choice is ampicillin.
C   Rheumatic chorea is a recognized sequela.
D   They are a cause of erysipelas.
E   Penicillin prophylaxis is indicated for 2 years following acute nephritis.

5.3.   Which of the following statements is/are true of meningococcal infections?
A   Penicillin is the drug of choice for chemoprophylaxis.
B   The meningococci can be cultured from haemorrhagic skin lesions.
C   Adrenal haemorrhage is a recognized complication.
D   Neurological sequelae are less likely following meningococcal meningitis than following other bacterial meningitis.
E   Blood cultures are rarely positive in the absence of skin lesions.

5.4. Bacterial infection is the primary cause of
A   impetigo contagiosa.
B   seborrhoeic dermatitis.
C   psoriasis.
D   toxic epidermal necrolysis (scalded skin syndrome).
E   molluscum contagiosum.

5.1. A E
Blood cultures are positive in supraglottic croup (the organism is *Haemophilus influenzae* b) and in 70% of cases of bacterial meningitis. Bronchiolitis is a viral infection. *Bordetella pertussis* is cultured by a nasopharyngeal swab. *Campylobacter* is isolated by stool culture.

5.2. A C D
Most respiratory infections in children under the age of 2 years are viral in origin. The treatment of choice for streptococcal sore throat is penicillin. Rheumatic chorea may occur long after streptococcal infection has resolved. Erysipelas, which has a well-defined erythematous margin, is due to streptococcal infection of dermis. Penicillin prophylaxis is not necessary following an attack of acute nephritis as second attacks are rare.

5.3. B C D
Penicillin-resistant meningococci have been isolated and hence contacts of meningococcal disease should be given rifampicin until culture results are obtained. The skin lesions contain the organisms. Adrenal haemorrhage occurs more commonly with septicaemia and shock. If meningococcal meningitis is diagnosed early, neurological sequelae are less common than after other forms of meningitis. Blood cultures are positive in most cases even in the absence of skin lesions.

5.4. A D
Impetigo is caused by streptococcal and staphylococcal infections. Toxic epidermal necrolysis is a complication of staphylococcal infection. The aetiology of seborrhoeic dermatitis and psoriasis is not known. Molluscum contagiosum is caused by a virus.

5.5. Which of the following statements is/are true of pertussis (whooping cough)?

A Immunization is effective in preventing this disease in over 95% of people.

B Immunization of premature infants in good health should be carried out 2 months after birth.

C Erythromycin has been shown to inhibit the growth of the aetiological agent *in vitro*.

D Children under the age of 3 months are not at risk from the disease.

E The incidence of permanent neurological complications from immunization is less than 0.1%.

5.6. In which of the following conditions is pertussis immunization contraindicated in a 2-month-old infant?

A Baby exhibited neurological abnormalities in the neonatal period.

B History of epilepsy in close relatives secondary to brain injury.

C Family history of eczema.

D Family history of cystic fibrosis.

E Temperature of 38.5°C on routine examination at time of presentation for immunization.

5.7. Whooping cough

A does not occur in the neonate if the mother has been previously immunized.

B is more common in preschool than older children.

C is contracted by droplet infection.

D occurs around 21 days after exposure.

E starts with a paroxysmal cough.

5.8. Which of the following statements is/are true of tuberculosis infection?

A A 2-year-old Australian born child with positive tuberculin test who has no clinical disease requires antituberculous treatment.

B BCG immunization has been proven to protect against miliary disease.

C Atypical mycobacteria organisms usually cause pulmonary disease in childhood.

D Chemotherapy is necessary only for 3 months.

E Mortality rate from tuberculosis decreased significantly only when effective antituberculous drugs were introduced.

5.5. B C E

Newborn infants do not have transplacentally acquired immunity against pertussis and should be immunized as early as possible. Correct age is 2 months for both full-term and premature infants. Erythromycin has been shown to inhibit the growth of the organism *in vitro*. The incidence of permanent neurological complications is less than 1 in 150 000 cases.

5.6. E

An acute illness (high fever) is a contraindication for immunization. None of the other conditions mentioned is an absolute contraindication for pertussis immunization.

5.7. B C

Newborn infants do not have transplacentally acquired immunity against whooping cough. The incubation period of pertussis is 6–14 days and it is spread by droplet infection. The illness starts with a catarrhal stage which consists of rhinorrhoea, conjunctival injection, mild cough, wheezing and a low-grade fever. The incidence is highest in children under 5 years of age and 30% of cases occur in infants less than 6 months of age. Mortality is greatest in infants under 1 year of age.

5.8. A B

Tuberculosis is rare in children born in Australia and a positive tuberculin test indicates that the child has been exposed to the tubercle bacillus. As there is a risk of generalized disease, treatment is indicated. BCG immunization results in primary infection which prevents generalized disease on reinfection. Atypical mycobacteria usually cause lymphadenitis. A 3-month course of chemotherapy for tuberculous infection is inadequate. Most patients require treatment for 6 months or longer. Mortality rates from tuberculosis decreased with improvement in housing and nutrition which decreased the spread of disease.

5.9. Which of the following statements about primary tuberculosis is/are correct?

A   The primary focus in the lung usually cavitates.

B   Symptoms from primary tuberculosis mostly arise from enlargement of the draining lymph nodes.

C   Some degree of blood-borne dissemination occurs with most cases of primary tuberculosis.

D   Sputum positive for acid-fast bacilli (AFB) is required before making a diagnosis of primary tuberculosis.

E   Most cases of miliary tuberculosis and tuberculous meningitis occur within 1 year of initial infection with tuberculosis.

5.10. The proper interpretation of a positive reaction to a tuberculin (Mantoux) test in a 9-year-old child is that the patient is

A   suffering from active tuberculosis.

B   immune to invasion by the tubercle bacillus.

C   susceptible to invasion by the tubercle bacillus.

D   in need of BCG vaccination.

E   sensitive to tuberculo-protein.

5.11. A child of 8 years has had a fever of 40°C (104°F) for 2 days. The tonsils are enlarged and inflamed and partly covered by a mucopurulent exudate. The cervical lymph nodes are enlarged and tender. Which of the following is/are true?

A   A negative Paul–Bunnell test would exclude glandular fever.

B   Hypertrophy of the lingual papillae and a confluent desquamating skin rash indicates haemolytic streptococcal infection.

C   If streptococci are grown from the throat swab, tetracycline is the treatment of choice in patients with penicillin allergy.

D   Palatal paralysis would indicate the need for immediate isolation.

E   Tonsillectomy should be advised following recovery.

5.12. Which of the following statements is/are true of Herpes simplex virus infection?

A   It can be transmitted sexually.

B   Primary infection is more severe than subsequent recurrence.

C   It is aggravated by exposure to the sun.

D   It often recurs in the same site.

E   It can be differentiated from other herpes viruses by electron microscopy.

5.9. B C E

The primary lesion in the lungs usually heals leaving a small scar. The enlarged lymph nodes cause symptoms by exerting pressure on bronchi. AFB are usually not isolated from the sputum in primary tuberculosis as there is no communication between the bronchi and the lung lesion. In primary tuberculosis the organisms are not localized to the site of infection and blood-borne dissemination occurs. Miliary tuberculosis and tuberculous meningitis can occur and usually do so within a year of initial infection.

5.10. E

A positive reaction to tuberculin indicates that the patient is sensitive to the tuberculo-protein, which means the patient has been infected previously by the tubercle bacillus. It does not indicate active disease, immunity to tuberculosis or susceptibility to infection with the tubercle bacillus. BCG vaccination is contraindicated in these individuals.

5.11. B D

It is not unusual for the Paul–Bunnell test to be negative in glandular fever in children. Specific assays for IgG and IgM antibodies to Epstein–Barr virus are more helpful in the diagnosis. Hypertrophy of the lingual papillae accompanied with a confluent desquamating rash suggests scarlet fever, which is caused by beta-haemolytic streptococcal infection. The treatment of choice for streptococcal infections in patients with penicillin allergy is erythromycin. In the presence of palatal paralysis with the history in the stem one should suspect diphtheria which requires isolation of the patient. There is no indication for tonsillectomy in this patient.

5.12. A B C D

Herpes simplex virus infection can be transmitted sexually; the type of virus identified most often in these cases is type 2. Approximately 85% of infections by herpes simplex virus are asymptomatic. The symptoms are more severe with primary infection. The virus remains latent in neural tissue and can be reactivated by stress or exposure to the sun, tending to recur at the same site. It is a DNA virus and cannot be distinguished from other herpes viruses by electron microscopy.

5.13. Which of the following statements is/are true of *Mycoplasma pneumoniae* respiratory tract infections in children?

A   They are diagnosed by demonstrating cold agglutinins in the blood.
B   They are a most common cause of pneumonia in school age children.
C   The organism is easily grown from sputum cultures.
D   The infections are associated with middle ear disease.
E   They are treated with erythromycin.

5.14. A boy aged 7 months presents with a temperature of 39°C and irritability for 3 days. On the 4th day the temperature subsides, a generalized macular rash appears and then he is not irritable. Which of the following statements is/are true?

A   This presentation is typical of morbilli.
B   A positive diagnosis will be made by viral cultures of throat swabbing.
C   A possible diagnosis will be made by CSF examination.
D   This presentation is typical of roseola infantum.
E   This presentation is typical of drug allergy.

5.15. A woman in the 3rd month of pregnancy was in contact the previous day with a known case of rubella. Which of the following statements regarding her serum immunoglobulins is/are true?

A   If rubella-specific IgG is found there is no risk to the fetus.
B   If rubella-specific IgG is not found, she should be immediately immunized with rubella vaccine.
C   If rubella-specific IgG is initially not found but present a week later, natural immunity has developed and the fetus will be protected.
D   If rubella-specific IgG is absent at the end of pregnancy and a healthy child is born no further action is necessary.
E   Demonstration of rubella-specific IgM one week later indicates recent infection.

5.16. Which of the following statements is/are true of infections with rubella virus?

A   Arthritis is a recognized complication.
B   The incubation period is 7–14 days.
C   Thrombocytopenia is a recognized complication.
D   Haemagglutination-inhibition antibodies are usually detected when a rash appears.
E   Haemagglutination-inhibition antibodies persist longer than complement fixation antibodies.

5.13. B D E

Although cold agglutinins are increased in *Mycoplasma pneumoniae* infections, they are not diagnostic and have been found in association with other viral respiratory infections. *M. pneumoniae* may cause pneumonia in any age group but it most commonly affects adolescents and young adults. It may cause upper respiratory disease and has been isolated from patients with otitis media. The organism cannot be isolated easily from the sputum. Complement fixation is the best serological test for the diagnosis. The organism is sensitive to erythromycin and tetracycline.

5.14. D

Fever and irritability followed by a macular rash when the temperature subsides is diagnostic of roseola infantum. Throat swab cultures for viruses and CSF examination are not helpful in making a diagnosis since the causative organism (HHV-6) is not readily isolated. The white cell count shows leukopenia with relative lymphocytosis. In measles the temperature rises when the rash appears.

5.15. A E

The presence of rubella-specific IgG indicates that the woman has been infected with rubella virus previously, and she is therefore unlikely to be reinfected. Her fetus is at no risk of developing congenital rubella. As rubella vaccine has been implicated in the aetiology of congenital rubella, rubella immunization is not recommended during pregnancy. The presence of rubella-specific IgG in a patient who was previously seronegative indicates recent infection, which means the fetus is at risk of developing infection. Absence of rubella-specific IgG at the end of pregnancy indicates that she is still at risk of developing rubella during subsequent pregnancies and needs to be protected against this by active immunization following delivery. A rise in rubella-specific IgM occurs soon after rubella infection.

5.16. A C E

The incubation period of rubella is 14–21 days. Clinical manifestations include polyarthritis (usually of the hands) and thrombocytopenia. Haemagglutination-inhibition antibody titres appear in the convalescent stage and persist longer than complement fixation antibodies.

5.17. Comparing measles (morbilli) with German measles (rubella), it is a characteristic of the former that
A   the incubation period is longer.
B   the temperature period is longer.
C   pre-exanthem symptoms are of longer duration.
D   Koplik's spots appear.
E   suboccipital glands are more prominent.

5.18. Which of the following is/are characteristic of measles?
A   Rhinitis.
B   Conjunctivitis.
C   Cough.
D   Enanthem.
E   Normal temperature when rash appears.

5.19. Which of the following statements is/are true of measles vaccine?
A   It is an inactivated virus.
B   The resulting protection lasts at least 5 years.
C   It is unaffected in efficacy by any pre-existing measles antibody which has been passively or transplacentally acquired.
D   It is more likely to provide protection when injected at age 15 months than at 9 months.
E   It is effective when given simultaneously with other immunizing agents.

5.20. Live measles vaccine should *not* be given to children
A   with leukaemia on chemotherapy.
B   on large doses of oral corticosteroids.
C   under the age of 3 months.
D   with egg allergy.
E   with HIV infection.

5.17. B C D

The incubation period of measles is 6–14 days; that of German measles is 14–21 days. The prodromal phase of rubella may go unnoticed whereas that of morbilli lasts 6–8 days and the fever persists and is maximum during the rash stage. Koplik spots are pathognomonic of measles whereas suboccipital glands are more prominent in German measles.

5.18. A B C D

Rhinitis, conjunctivitis, cough and enanthem (Koplik spots) are manifestations of the prodromal phase of measles. The fever rises when the rash appears.

5.19. B D E

Measles vaccine consists of a live virus and its immune effect lasts at least 5 years. When given at 9 months it is likely to be less effective because of the neutralization of the vaccine by maternally derived measles antibodies. The immunity will occur even when measles vaccine is given with other immunizing agents.

5.20. A B C

Live measles vaccine is contraindicated in patients who have immunosuppression, which includes those receiving chemotherapy or corticosteroids. However, experience has shown that it is safe in children with HIV infection and appears to offer protection to such children. Moreover, fatal episodes of measles have been reported in unimmunized children with HIV infection. It is not as effective if given to children under the age of 1 year and is not advised for use in children under the age of 3 months. Although anaphylaxis following egg ingestion is a contraindication to measles immunization, allergy by itself is not a contraindication.

5.21. Which of the following statements is/are true of chickenpox?

A   The patient is infective until all the scales have fallen.
B   Macules, papules, vesicles and scabs may be seen in different stages of development.
C   An intramuscular injection of human pooled gammaglobulin can modify the course of disease in contacts.
D   Encephalitis is a recognized complication.
E   It is a recognized cause of calcification in the lungs.

5.22. Mumps

A   can be prevented by active immunization.
B   has a 2–3 week incubation period.
C   rarely affects the testes before puberty.
D   is rarely complicated by meningitis.
E   can cause nerve deafness.

5.23. Which of the following statements is/are true of pin worm (*Enterobius vermicularis*) infestation in children?

A   It is a common cause of anaemia.
B   It can be transmitted directly from one child to another without an animal vector.
C   The pinworms migrate out through the anus to deposit their eggs on the perianal skin.
D   It is usually asymptomatic.
E   It is diagnosed by microscopy of stool specimen.

5.24. Which of the following statements is/are true concerning *Giardia lamblia* infestation in childhood?

A   Metronidazole is an appropriate therapeutic agent.
B   Stool microscopy is the most reliable diagnostic test.
C   It is a cause of intestinal disaccharide intolerance.
D   It does not occur in the first 4 weeks of life.
E   It is the cause of coeliac disease.

5.21. B D E
In chickenpox the patient is infective 2 days before and 7 days after the onset of the rash and until all lesions are crusted. The lesions may be at different stages of maturity, i.e. macules, papules, vesicles and scabs may be seen simultaneously. Complications include encephalitis, secondary bacterial infection, thrombocytopenia, haemorrhagic lesions leading to purpura fulminans, myocarditis, pericarditis, myositis, hepatitis, glomerulonephritis, arthritis and Reye syndrome. Primary varicella pneumonia may be complicated by pleurisy with effusion, and calcification in the lungs has been reported following chickenpox. Varicella contacts can be protected by injection of zoster immune globulin, large amounts of human pooled globulin administered intravenously, or by antiviral therapy.

5.22. A B C E
Mumps immunization is carried out at the same age as measles and rubella immunizations (15 months). The incubation period of mumps is 2–3 weeks. Orchitis and epididymitis is rare in prepubescent boys but is common (14–35%) in adolescents and adults. Approximately 30–40% of affected testes atrophy. Although impairment of fertility is estimated to be about 10%, absolute infertility is rare. Meningoencephalitis is the most frequent complication in childhood (more than 65% of children show pleocytosis of cerebrospinal fluid). Unilateral nerve deafness, may occur although the incidence is low (1 in 15 000). It is a leading cause of unilateral nerve deafness which may be transient or permanent.

5.23. B C D
Pinworm infestation does not cause anaemia. Infection occurs by ingesting the eggs which are usually carried on fingernails, clothing, bedding or housedust or by autoinfection. The eggs are deposited by the worm on the perianal skin which results in perianal irritation and induces scratching, although in the majority of cases there are no symptoms. Diagnosis is made by demonstrating the eggs on adhesive tape.

5.24. A C
Giardia lamblia infestation is best diagnosed by duodenal biopsy and examination of a wet preparation of intestinal mucosa. It causes lactose intolerance and responds to treatment with metronidazole. It can occur at any age and is not the cause of coeliac disease, which is due to gluten enteropathy.

5.25. Toxoplasmosis is
A   a bacterial disease.
B   a cause of lymphadenitis.
C   usually lethal in man.
D   due to an organism that can cross the placental barrier.
E   resistant to treatment with sulphonamides.

5.26. In the infant of a woman with HIV infection which of the following is/are correct?
A   Transmission of HIV infection may take place during parturition.
B   Transmission of HIV infection during breast feeding has not been reported.
C   The risk of HIV infection in the infant is greater than 80%.
D   Failure to thrive may be the presenting symptom.
E   Diagnosis of HIV in the newborn infant usually cannot be made with routinely available serological tests.

5.27. Which of the following is/are common presentations of infants with HIV infection?
A   Failure to thrive.
B   Developmental delay.
C   Chronic diarrhoea.
D   Glandular fever-like illness.
E   Recurrent bacterial pneumonia.

5.28. Immunoglobulin G (IgG)
A   does not cross the placenta.
B   is the main immunoglobulin of external secretions.
C   is secreted by macrophages.
D   is the predominant serum immunoglobulin.
E   provides immunity against *Mycobacterium tuberculosis*.

5.25. B D
Toxoplasmosis is caused by *Toxoplasma gondii*, which is a coccidian protozoan. It is an intracellular parasite which can multiply in all tissues of mammals and birds. Infection may be congenital, when it may manifest like any other congenital infection, or acquired. The latter may be asymptomatic or present with malaise, fever, myalgia, maculopapular rash, localized or generalized lymphadenopathy, hepatomegaly, encephalitis, pneumonia, myocarditis and choroidoretinitis. Although the organism is sensitive to sulphonamides, a combination of pyrimethamine and sulphonamides is superior.

5.26. A D E
Transmission of HIV infection from mother to infant can occur at birth through maternal blood and/or secretions. Infection has been reported to be acquired through breast milk. However, maternal HIV infection is not an absolute contraindication for breast feeding. Vertical transmission *in utero* occurs in 15–40% of cases. Common presentations in infancy include failure to thrive, lymphoid interstitial hyperplasia, opportunistic and bacterial infections, diarrhoea, hepatosplenomegaly and lymphadenopathy. Diagnosis in the newborn is difficult because HIV antibodies cross the placenta readily and HIV antigen testing is insensitive.

5.27. A B C E
Infants with HIV infection may fail to thrive due to chronic diarrhoea and recurrent infections as a result of immune deficiency. They may be developmentally delayed. A febrile illness with glandular enlargement is not a feature of HIV infection in infants.

5.28. D
IgG crosses the placenta, and is the predominant serum immunoglobulin. It does not provide immunity against *Mycobacterium tuberculosis*. It is secreted by plasma cells which differentiate from B cells. The main immunoglobulin in external secretions is IgA.

5.29. In which of the following situations would you advise vaccination?

A   Triple antigen to a well, premature infant at the age of 2 months.

B   Sabin vaccination in a child with recurrent or persistent *Candida* infection of the skin and/or mucous membranes.

C   Hyperimmune gammaglobulin with hepatitis B vaccine to a newborn infant whose mother is hepatitis B surface antigen-positive.

D   Measles vaccine to a 4-year-old child recently exposed to measles.

E   Tetanus toxoid for a 2-year-old child with a penetrating wound in the foot caused by a builder's nail, who is up to date with triple antigen vaccination.

5.30. Which of the following statements is/are true?

A   Pertussis vaccine should not be given to wheezing babies.

B   Sabin vaccine should not be given to immunosuppressed infants.

C   Atopy is not a contraindication to measles vaccination.

D   Skin reactions at the site of injection are not a contraindication to continue DPT immunization.

E   Diphtheria and tetanus antitoxin levels persist for 10 years or more in adequately immunized persons.

5.31. Which of the following statements is/are true?

A   Triple antigen is given by subcutaneous injection.

B   A full course of immunization is adequate even if 3–4 months elapse between the first and second injections.

C   Sabin vaccine can be administered intramuscularly if the child vomits following oral administration.

D   Intraventricular haemorrhage in the newborn is not a contraindication for triple vaccine.

E   Triple vaccine should be stored in the freezer compartment of the refrigerator.

5.32. Which of the following statements is/are correct?

A   Macrophages are derived from precursor cells in the bone marrow.

B   B lymphocytes are the precursors of plasma cells.

C   T lymphocytes are the precursors of immunoglobulin-forming cells.

D   T lymphocytes are responsible for rejecting grafts.

E   The plasma cells produce transfer factor.

5.29. A C D
Premature infants should be offered triple antigen at the chronological age of 2 months (i.e. the same as full-term infants). Recurrent and persistent *Candida* infection suggests disturbance of the T-cell function and is a contraindication for administration of live vaccine such as Sabin. Hepatitis B surface antigen-positive mothers excrete the virus in all body secretions (milk, saliva) and are likely to infect their newborn infants, especially if e antigen positive. This can be prevented by administration of hyperimmune gammaglobulin. Measles vaccine will provide adequate protection if given soon after exposure to measles. Another tetanus toxoid injection is not required because immunity to tetanus following inoculation lasts 5–10 years.

5.30. B C D E
There is no contraindication for giving pertussis vaccine to wheezing babies or giving measles vaccination to atopic children. Live vaccines (which include Sabin) are contraindicated for immunosuppressed infants as they may develop clinical disease. DPT immunization may be completed in infants with localized skin reactions. In severe cases prophylactic administration of antihistamines is indicated. After immunization diphtheria and tetanus antitoxins persist for 10 years or more.

5.31. B D
Triple antigen is given by deep intramuscular injection and is effective even if 3–4 months lapse between the first and second injections. Sabin vaccine is administered orally. Following administration there is subclinical enteral infection which is necessary to stimulate immunity. Intraventricular haemorrhage in the newborn is not a contraindication to immunization with triple antigen (including pertussis vaccine). The vaccine is stored in the non-freezer part of the refrigerator.

5.32. A B D
The marrow-derived lymphocytes (B cells) are the precursors of plasma cells and immunoglobulin-forming cells. Macrophages are derived from the myeloid series in the bone marrow. The thymus-derived lymphocytes (T cells) are the principal cells responsible for rejecting grafts. They also protect against viral infections and produce cytokines, including interferon gamma and transfer factor.

5.33. Which of the following is/are correct?
A   Allergen-induced reactions are mediated via IgE bound to mucosal eosinophils.
B   Newborn infants of mothers allergic to milk may be milk-sensitive due to transplacental transfer of specific IgE antibody.
C   A reduced level of the fourth component of complement (C4) may be useful in the diagnosis of hereditary angioedema.
D   IgE antibodies help in the elimination of parasites.
E   Raised IgA levels in cord blood indicate congenital infection.

5.34. For which of the following diseases can a diagnosis be made by flow cytometric analysis of lymphocyte subsets?
A   X-linked hypogammaglobulinaemia (XLH).
B   Severe combined immunodeficiency (SCID).
C   diGeorgé anomaly (DGA).
D   Leukocyte adhesion defect (LAD).
E   Ataxia telangiectasia (AT).

5.35. Which of the following statements is/are correct?
A T_{H1} cells produce interleukin 2 and interferon gamma.
B T_{H1} cells promote cell mediated immunity.
C T_{H2} cells secrete interleukins 4 and 5.
D   Interleukin 4 production promotes the switching of B cells to IgE production.
E   Interleukin 5 promotes eosinophil growth and differentiation.

5.33. C D

Immediate hypersensitivity reactions are mediated by IgE bound to basophils and mast cells. Allergens may induce delayed hypersensitivity reactions. Macrophages coated with IgE anti-parasite immune complexes are particularly effective in eliminating parasitic infestations. Only IgG is transferred transplacentally. Raised IgA levels in cord blood indicate contamination of cord blood with maternal blood. Cord blood IgM is raised in infants with congenital infections. C4 levels are reduced in hereditary angioedema.

5.34. A B D

B cells are characteristically absent in XLH but are present, though dysfunctional, in acquired hypogammaglobulinaemia. T cell numbers are markedly reduced in SCID; B cells may be either absent or present. In DGA lymphocyte abnormalities may be quite subtle. In LAD the absence of the CD18–CD11b complex on phagocytic cells is probably of most significance, though the defective gene is that of CD18, and other CD18-dependent structures (CD18-CD11a or LFA_1) are absent from lymphocytes. There are no characteristic abnormalities in lymphocyte surface markers in AT.

5.35. A B C D E

T_{H1} cells produce interleukin 2 and interferon-γ. They promote cell-mediated immunity including delayed hypersensitivity. T_{H2} cells secrete interleukins 4 and 5. Interleukin 4 promotes IgE production by stimulating B cell isotype switching and interleukin 5 promotes eosinophil growth and differentiation. Interleukin 4 also favours maturation of T cells into T_{H2}-type cells while interferon-γ favours T_{H1} production (positive feedback mechanisms). The T_{H2} response is believed to be prominent in allergic reactions.

6 Gastrointestinal system

6.1. Swelling of the gums is significantly associated with which of the following conditions?
A   Scurvy.
B   Acute lymphoblastic leukaemia.
C   Hypothyroidism.
D   Phenytoin therapy.
E   Poor orodental hygiene.

6.2. Which of the following statements is/are true of gastro-oesophageal reflux?
A   It is associated with apnoeic spells.
B   It may present with wheezing.
C   It usually causes projectile vomiting.
D   Barium swallow and radiological screening is a reliable method of establishing a diagnosis.
E   It may cause failure to thrive.

6.3. Which of the following statements is/are correct of gastro-oesophageal reflux in infancy?
A   Iron deficiency anaemia may be the presenting symptom.
B   Aspiration pneumonia is a complication.
C   The condition tends to improve spontaneously by 6–8 months of age.
D   It can be treated with cisapride.
E   It is often associated with cerebral palsy.

6.4. The symptoms and clinical findings in a newborn with oesophageal atresia *without fistula* include
A   'mucusy' at birth.
B   cyanotic spells.
C   abdominal distension.
D   aspiration of gastric content if nursed supine.
E   meconium containing no hair.

6.1. A D E

Swelling of the gums occurs in scurvy due to bleeding (only if teeth have erupted), gum hypertrophy due to phenytoin therapy and infection due to poor oro-dental hygiene. It is not a feature of acute lymphoblastic leukaemia or hypothyroidism.

6.2. A B E

The apnoeic attacks are caused by reflex action in response to acid in the oesophagus. Aspiration of the gastric contents will result in aspiration pneumonia and wheezing. Vomiting is usually effortless. Failure to thrive will result if the vomiting is persistent and in large amounts. As the reflux may be intermittent, barium swallow and radiological screening will not establish the diagnosis as reliably as prolonged oesophageal pH probe assessment.

6.3. A B C D E

In gastro-oesophageal reflux iron deficiency anaemia occurs due to reflux oesophagitis and bleeding. Aspiration pneumonia is due to the aspiration of stomach contents into the lungs. It tends to improve when the child adopts a sitting posture. Vomiting is usually effortless. Cisapride improves oesophageal sphincter tone and gastric motility which alleviate the vomiting. The incidence is increased in patients with cerebral palsy.

6.4. A B E

The infant is 'mucusy' at birth because it is unable to swallow its saliva. Cyanotic spells occur due to the aspiration of the saliva into the trachea. Meconium does not contain hair as the fetus is unable to swallow amniotic fluid. Abdominal distension and aspiration of gastric contents cannot take place because there is no fistula between the oesophagus and trachea.

6.5. A 5-week-old infant presents with projectile vomiting of increasing severity for 10 days. He appears moderately dehydrated. The probable laboratory findings would be

A   elevated blood pH.
B   increased serum chloride.
C   increased serum bicarbonate level.
D   decreased urinary potassium level.
E   low serum potassium level.

6.6. Which of the following statements is/are true of infantile hypertrophic pyloric stenosis?

A   The narrowing of the lumen is principally due to hypertrophy of the longitudinal muscular layer.
B   The onset is rare before the age of 1 week
C   The infant takes feeds well.
D   The vomitus usually contains bile.
E   Small green frequent stools do not exclude the diagnosis.

6.7. Which of the following statements is/are correct?

A   Enteropeptidase (enterokinase) deficiency causes malabsorption.
B   Amylase deficiency usually causes diarrhoea.
C   Cholestatic disorders of the liver give rise to fat globules in the stools.
D   Massive diarrhoea can occur with neuroblastoma.
E   The peripheral neuritis associated with abetalipoproteinaemia is due to vitamin A deficiency.

6.8. Which of the following statements is/are true of intestinal sugar intolerance?

A   Hereditary lactose intolerance usually presents before the age of 2 years.
B   Hereditary glucose/galactose malabsorption can be treated by a lactose-free soya formula.
C   Infants can develop disaccharide intolerance following infectious diarrhoea.
D   Lactose intolerance can be diagnosed by measuring expired breath hydrogen.
E   Small bowel bacterial overgrowth can present with symptoms of sugar intolerance.

6.5. A C E

Projectile vomiting of increasing severity in a 5-week-old infant is most likely to be due to pyloric stenosis, which would result in loss of gastric fluid containing hydrochloric acid and potassium. This will result in raised blood pH, a fall in serum chloride and increased serum bicarbonate level. In order to maintain a normal pH, renal tubules will reabsorb hydrogen ions at the expense of excreting potassium ions in the urine, resulting in an increased urinary potassium loss in spite of low serum potassium level.

6.6. B C E

In infantile hypertrophic pyloric stenosis the narrowing of the lumen is due to hypertrophy of the circular muscular layer. The onset is usually in the second to third week of life. As the stomach remains empty, the infant is hungry and feeds readily. The vomitus usually consists of gastric contents and contains no bile. The infant may have small green frequent stools which also occur in other conditions with starvation.

6.7. A C D

Enteropeptidase converts trypsinogen to trypsin as well as procolipase to colipase, which activates lipase. Insufficiency causes malabsorption. Although starch contains many molecules of carbohydrate it has a low osmotic effect and therefore malabsorption due to amylase deficiency does not usually cause diarrhoea. Fat globules are found in the stools as fat remains insoluble in water (and is not absorbed) in the absence of bile salts. Ten percent of neuroblastomas secrete vasoactive intestinal peptide (VIP) which causes secretory diarrhoea. Peripheral neuritis in abetalipoproteinaemia is due to vitamin E malabsorption.

6.8. C D E

The onset of hereditary permanent lactose deficiency very rarely occurs before the age of 2 years but increases in frequency through childhood. Soya formulae usually contain sucrose or glucose polymer which, when hydrolysed, liberates glucose which cannot be absorbed in individuals with hereditary glucose–galactose malabsorption. Following infectious diarrhoea most infants develop lactose intolerance; some may also develop sucrose intolerance. In lactose intolerance hydrogen appears late in the breath as it is liberated from the disaccharide by the colonic bacteria. Bacterial overgrowth of the small bowel is associated with mucosal injury and depression of disaccharide enzyme levels, which presents as sugar intolerance.

114

6.9. In watery diarrhoea due to lactose intolerance
A   Clinistix will detect the lactose in the stool.
B   the stools will usually change blue litmus paper red.
C   the diarrhoea will be fermentative (excess gas produced).
D   the findings of 0.25% sugar in the stool strongly supports the diagnosis.
E   for testing the stool is best collected off a nappy or bed sheet.

6.10. Chronic diarrhoea may be the presenting symptom of
A   cystic fibrosis.
B   lactose intolerance.
C   excessive consumption of fruit juices and cordials.
D   intestinal lymphangiectasia.
E   coeliac disease.

6.11. Which of the following statements is/are correct of coeliac disease?
A   The clinical disease may be initiated by a diet high in rye cereal.
B   Antigliandin IgA levels can be reliably used in establishing the diagnosis.
C   The condition has a self-limiting course and usually abates in late childhood.
D   The condition is diagnosed by assessing the clinical response to a gluten-free diet.
E   Typically during childhood the condition is associated with marked irritability.

6.12. Which of the following statements is/are correct in regard to coeliac disease?
A   The gluten-free diet should be continued throughout life.
B   There is an increased incidence in close relatives of affected children.
C   The malabsorption is due to pancreatic deficiency.
D   It is diagnosed on the basis of symptomatic response to a gluten-free diet.
E   Clinical onset is usually recognizable by 4 months of age.

6.9. B C

Clinistix is specific for glucose and hence will not detect lactose. The stools are acid and will therefore turn litmus paper from blue to red. Lactose in the stool is fermented by gut organisms. It is not uncommon for normal stools to contain up to 0.25% sugar. It is important to obtain the liquid part of the stool for testing and therefore it is better to collect it on a plastic sheet or obtain it by passing a soft rubber catheter into the rectum.

6.10. A B C D E

Chronic diarrhoea occurs in cystic fibrosis because of lack of pancreatic enzymes and in lactose intolerance because of high osmolarity of unabsorbed sugars. Fruit juices, cordials and lollies contain fructose and/or sorbitol which are poorly absorbed and cause osmotic diarrhoea. In coeliac disease the diarrhoea is due to malabsorption following damage to the intestinal villi and epithelial cells. In intestinal lymphangiestasia fat malabsorption and albumin loss cause diarrhoea.

6.11. A E

Coeliac disease is caused by gluten (which is present in wheat, rye, barley and oats). Antigliadin IgA levels may be low because serum IgA deficiency is found commonly in coeliac disease; antigliadin IgA cannot, therefore, be produced. Furthermore false high antigliadin IgA levels are seen in normal individuals. It is a lifelong disease and is diagnosed by small bowel biopsy prior to introducing a gluten-free diet. One of the presenting symptoms in childhood is irritability.

6.12. A B

In coeliac disease gluten sensitivity is permanent and increases the risk of malignancy. The gluten-free diet should therefore be continued throughout life. The condition is familial and pancreatic dysfunction is minimal. Diagnosis is based on demonstrating villous atrophy, regeneration of the villi following a gluten-free diet and recurrence of villous atrophy after reintroduction of gluten. Clinical onset does not occur until some time after the introduction of gluten in the diet.

6.13. In Crohn's disease of childhood
A the stomach and duodenum may be involved.
B diarrhoea with blood and mucus is a characteristic early symptom.
C growth retardation is a characteristic feature.
D surgical resection of the affected gut is curative.
E fever of unknown origin may be the presenting symptom.

6.14. Intussusception in childhood
A may undergo spontaneous cure.
B has, as the earliest sign, the passage of redcurrant jelly stools.
C has a peak incidence in the first 3 months of life.
D requires operative reduction in the majority of cases.
E may be initiated by a Meckel's diverticulum.

6.15. Intussusception in childhood is
A most common in infants aged 6–9 months.
B a self-limited condition.
C more common in fat babies.
D generally associated with an umbilical hernia.
E a recognized complication of Henoch–Schönlein purpura.

6.16. The treatment of a central umbilical hernia in a 4-month-old infant is
A immediate surgical repair.
B surgical repair at the age of 8 months.
C application of a coin with adhesive tape.
D reassurance of the mother.
E none of the above.

6.17. Inguinal hernias
A are more common than femoral hernias.
B are more common in premature infants.
C usually present with pain in the groin.
D require an early elective operation.
E require herniorrhaphy in children.

6.13. A C E

As in adults, Crohn's disease in childhood affects the terminal ileum most frequently, though in most cases the stomach and duodenum show granulomas on microscopy as the disease progresses. Growth retardation and fever of unknown origin are the common presenting symptoms; diarrhoea with blood and mucus is a late symptom. Surgical resection of the gut is not recommended unless there are complications such as perforation or intestinal obstruction.

6.14. A E

Intussusception may undergo spontaneous cure and may be started by a Meckel's diverticulum, though this is rare. Blood and mucus are late signs and may not appear at all. The peak incidence is at 6–8 months, usually after weaning. Barium or air enema will confirm the diagnosis and can be used to reduce the intussusception in the majority of cases.

6.15. A C E

Intussusception typically occurs in well infants soon after weaning and progresses to gangrene of the bowel and shock. It has no association with umbilical hernias. In Henoch–Schönlein purpura the lead point is an intramural haematoma.

6.16. D

As the majority of umbilical hernias resolve spontaneously, the mother needs reassurance. If the problem persists beyond the age of 2 years the child may need an operation.

6.17. A B D

Femoral hernias are extremely rare in children. The incidence of inguinal hernias in premature infants is at least three times that in full-term infants. Inguinal hernias rarely cause pain: pain in the groin is much more likely to represent hip disease than hernia. Surgical repair should be carried out as soon as possible as inguinal hernias in children tend to strangulate. Repair is carried out by high ligation of the sac. When a large internal inguinal ring exists, however, it is narrowed.

6.18. Which of the following statements related to infantile inguinal hernia is/are correct?

A   Left-sided hernia is more common than right-sided hernia.

B   Inguinal hernia in a phenotypically female infant may contain testis.

C   The majority are direct.

D   An inguinal hernia associated with an undescended testis should be operated only when the neonate has reached the age suitable for orchidopexy.

E   The chance of bilateral hernias in a male infant is higher if he presents with a left rather than right hernia.

6.19. Which of the following statements is/are true of diarrhoea and vomiting in infants?

A   Approximately 60% of cases in winter months in temperate climates are due to rotavirus.

B   It may be the presenting feature of urinary tract infection.

C   Crampy abdominal pain is a prominent feature of *Campylobacter* infections.

D   A normal potassium in serum indicates that potassium chloride is not needed in the intravenous fluids.

E   Lactose intolerance is a common sequel in infants.

6.20. Which of the following methods of management would you consider appropriate for gastroenteritis?

A   An electrolyte mixture containing 2% glucose for fluid replacement of a 2-year-old infant with 3–5% dehydration.

B   An electrolyte mixture containing 2% lactose for fluid replacement in an infant with mild rotavirus gastroenteritis.

C   Continuation of breast feeding with water between feeds for a 3-month-old baby with mild dehydration and watery diarrhoea containing more than 2% reducing sugars.

D   A normal diet for a 3-year-old child with mild diarrhoea.

E   A low lactose (lactose-hydrolysed milk-based) diet for a 7-month-old breast-fed infant with 8% dehydration and reducing sugar-positive fluid diarrhoea.

6.18. B E

In about 1% of phenotypically female infants the hernia may contain a testis. Such infants do not have a uterus and laparotomy reveals the absence of internal genital organs. Further investigations will reveal that the infant has testicular feminization syndrome. Inguinal hernias are indirect, i.e. they follow the track of the descent of the testis, and should be operated on as soon as possible after presentation as they are likely to strangulate. As the right testis descends after the left testis it is more likely that a hernia will also be present on the right side if one is present on the left. This also accounts for the higher incidence of right-sided inguinal hernias.

6.19. A B C E

Rotavirus is the most common organism causing gastroenteritis in winter months. Any parenteral infection (including urinary tract infection) in infants can present with diarrhoea. In *Campylobacter* infections the prominent symptoms are crampy abdominal pain and blood in stools. In gastroenteritis there is a net loss of potassium and intravenous fluids should provide potassium. Following gastroenteritis there is destruction of the brush border of the small intestine which results in lactase deficiency and lactose intolerance for a period of 1–4 weeks.

6.20. A C D

Glucose in electrolyte solution helps in absorption of the fluid and electrolytes. Patients with gastroenteritis have lactose intolerance and an electrolyte mixture containing lactose will, therefore, aggravate the problem. Breast-fed infants should continue receiving breast milk (after rehydration if necessary) as it is well tolerated and will provide protective IgA antibodies. There is no need to change the diet in a 3-year-old with mild diarrhoea. Patients with 8% dehydration would need intravenous fluids.

6.21. Which of the following statements regarding rotavirus diarrhoea in infants is/are correct?

A   Its incubation period is 48–72 h.
B   Fever is a prominent feature.
C   Respiratory symptoms are present in one-third to one-quarter of patients.
D   Glucose-stimulated sodium transport is impaired.
E   Intracellular cyclic AMP levels are normal.

6.22. Which of the following statements is/are true of gastroenteritis?

A   'Lomotil' (diphenoxylate and atropine mixture) will reduce the duration of the illness.
B   An infant under the age of 1 month should be admitted to hospital even though he may have mild symptoms.
C   Lactose intolerance, if present, is likely to be transient.
D   When due to *Salmonella typhimurium* it should be treated with amoxycillin or co-trimoxazole.
E   Anti-emetics are not recommended for children under the age of 5 years.

6.23. Recurrent abdominal pain is a recognized feature of

A   thread worm infestation.
B   Crohn's disease.
C   cystic fibrosis.
D   constipation.
E   emotional stress.

6.24. Which of the following statements is/are true of acute appendicitis in childhood?

A   Children over 8 years present with signs and symptoms similar to adults.
B   The initial presentation in a child under 4 is often generalized peritonitis.
C   A normal white cell count rules out the diagnosis.
D   Presence of urinary symptoms excludes the diagnosis.
E   Infants prefer to lie with hips flexed.

6.21. A B C D E
The incubation period of rotavirus diarrhoea is very short (48–72 h). Fever and respiratory symptoms are prominent and the patient has profuse watery diarrhoea due to impairment of glucose and glucose-stimulated sodium transport, but intracellular cyclic AMP levels are normal.

6.22. B C E
Antiemetic and antidiarrhoeal medications have no place in the treatment of gastroenteritis in infants and may cause harm by further disturbing gut motility or causing dystonic reactions. Neonates require admission to hospital because of the risk of rapid deterioration and dehydration. Lactose intolerance is due to the reduction in disaccharide enzyme activity which follows injury to the small intestine epithelial cells and their microvilli. *Salmonella* enteritis in infants is self-limiting. Administration of antibiotics results in prolongation of the period of clinical disease and the carrier stage.

6.23. B C D E
Thread worm infestation is either asymptomatic or causes perineal irritation or pruritis. Although the early symptoms of Crohn's disease are non-specific (fever, weight loss), in time most children develop crampy abdominal pain and diarrhoea. In cystic fibrosis the abdominal pain is due to sub-acute intestinal obstruction (meconium ileus equivalents). Recurrent abdominal pain due to constipation occurs after meals. Emotional stress is the most common cause of recurrent abdominal pain in a child with no physical signs. Such children also have leg pains and go on to develop tension headaches.

6.24. A B E
Pain is invariably present in appendicitis. The infant is irritable and has a tendency to lie quietly with hips flexed. Children under 5 years develop generalized peritonitis. Localized peritonitis is the usual presentation in older children and adults. The white cell count may be normal. Urinary symptoms occur as a result of inflamed appendix lying over the ureter.

6.25. In which of the following conditions are fat droplets likely to be observed in the faeces?

A Coeliac disease.
B Sucrase-isomaltase deficiency.
C Intestinal lymphangiectasia.
D Pancreatic achylia (Schwachman's syndrome).
E Biliary atresia.

6.26. Which of the following statements is/are true?

A Six to eight watery, yellow stools daily with curds are within the normal range for breast-fed infants.
B Breast-fed infants who pass no stools for 3 days require a laxative.
C The presence of 0.5% lactose in stools of a breast-fed baby usually requires no treatment.
D Breast-fed babies do not develop cows' milk allergy.
E The presence of greenish-grey stools in a bottle-fed (commercial formula) baby requires further laboratory investigations.

6.27. Acute anal fissure is

A associated with pain on defaecation.
B a cause of bright blood streaks on surface of motion.
C a recognized feature of Crohn's disease.
D best treated by surgical excision.
E associated with constipation.

6.28. Which of the following statements is/are true of Hirschsprung's disease?

A The rectum is usually empty.
B The symptoms may be mild while the child is fully breast-fed.
C The dilated portion of the gut shows absence of parasympathetic ganglia.
D The incidence is higher in infants who have meconium plugs at birth.
E It is rarely present in premature infants.

6.25. D E

In pancreatic achylia there is deficiency of pancreatic enzymes including lipase, which results in failure of digestion of fat. In biliary atresia fat droplets appear in the stool because the process of absorbing whole fats by emulsification is inhibited. In coeliac disease and intestinal lymphangiectasia there are no fat droplets in stools, although steatorrhoea is present, as fat is digested by pancreatic lipase to triglycerides and glycerol.

6.26. A C

It is normal for breast-fed infants to pass 6–8 stools a day or 1 stool in a week. Their stools contain up to 0.5% lactose. Breast-fed infants can develop cows' milk allergy because of the passage of cows' milk protein through breast milk. Greenish-grey stools in bottle-fed babies are due to the iron in the formula.

6.27. A B C E

Acute anal fissure is painful and causes spasm of the anal sphincter which results in pain on defaecation. The problem usually starts with constipation and may perpetuate it. The stools are blood streaked as bleeding occurs during defaecation. Anal fissure is a common complication of Crohn's disease. Surgical excision is rarely required.

6.28. A B D E

In Hirschsprung's disease, because of lack of peristalsis, the aganglionic segment is narrow and empty and the neurologically normal proximal portion of the gut is dilated. The condition may present as a meconium plug at birth. It has been shown to be rare in premature infants. Low levels of residues in breast milk may account for the delay in onset of symptoms.

6.29. Which of the following is/are associated with constipation?

A   Anal fissure
B   Hirschsprung's disease.
C   Hyperparathyroidism.
D   Hypothyroidism.
E   Faecal soiling.

6.30. A 2-month-old breast-fed infant is brought to see you because of persistent jaundice since birth. His stools are pale and his urine is highly coloured. Urine shows presence of bile but no urobilin. Which of the following is/are possible diagnosis/es?

A   Hypothyroidism.
B   Congenital viral infection.
C   Hereditary spherocytosis.
D   Congenital biliary atresia.
E   Breast milk jaundice.

6.31. Which of the following statements regarding hepatitis B is/are true?

A   It may be acquired by the faecal–oral route.
B   Hepatitis B surface antigen can usually be identified in the first week of the illness.
C   Persistence of antigenaemia for more than 3 months after the acute attack may be associated with chronic liver disease.
D   The incubation period is 4 weeks.
E   Newborn infants whose mothers have hepatitis B surface antibodies require hyperimmune gammaglobulin for prophylaxis.

6.29. A B C D E

In constipation, anal fissure may be caused by the hard stool. The anal fissure can perpetuate constipation by spasm of the anal sphincter due to pain. The principal manifestations of Hirschsprung's disease are intestinal obstruction and constipation. Rectal examination shows an empty anal canal. Faecal soiling occurs in constipation because irritation of the bowel mucosa by the hard stool causes secretion of mucus, which tracks down the gut wall. Hypercalcaemia, including that observed in hyperparathyrodism, is a recognized cause of constipation. Hypothyroidism slows gut peristalsis.

6.30. B D

This patient has obstructive jaundice, which occurs in congenital viral infections and congenital biliary atresia. The jaundice of hypothyroidism, hereditary spherocytosis and breast milk is not obstructive.

6.31. A B C

Although commonly acquired by injection of contaminated body fluids, hepatitis B can be acquired by the faecal–oral route. Hepatitis B surface antigen can be identified in serum soon after the onset of illness. Its persistence leads to chronic liver disease. The disease has an incubation period of more than 6 weeks. The presence of surface antibodies indicates that the person has immunity to hepatitis B. Such persons are not carriers (or infective) and their contacts do not require passive immunization.

7 Respiratory system

7.1. Airways beyond the terminal brochiole
A   contain no cartilage.
B   contribute largely to total airway resistance.
C   are structurally supported by the elastic network of the lung.
D   are influenced in calibre by pleural pressure changes.
E   cause wheezing if obstructed.

7.2. Arterial hypoxaemia in acute asthma
A   may be unchanged despite improvement in FEV_1 in the acute phase.
B   is usually associated with hypercapnia.
C   may occur in the absence of rhonchi on auscultation.
D   may worsen after intravenous aminophylline.
E   need not be associated with cyanosis.

7.3. Pulmonary oedema occurs in which of the following?
A   Smoke inhalation in a fire.
B   Transfusion reaction.
C   Sea water drowning.
D   Heart failure complicating isolated pulmonary stenosis.
E   Pneumonia.

7.4. Pulmonary function tests in a child with moderately severe asthma are likely to show
A   increased vital capacity.
B   increased functional residual capacity.
C   normal timed vital capacity (FEV_1).
D   increased lung elastic recoil.
E   increased total lung capacity.

7.1. A C D
Airways contain cartilage down to generation 16 (terminal bronchiole). Beyond that part the airways are held patent by negative pleural pressure and by the integrity of the perialveolar elastic network. These peripheral airways, because of their enormous total cross-sectional area, contribute little to total airways resistance. As the gas velocity is very low, wheezing is not heard in peripheral airway obstruction.

7.2. C D E
Improvement in FEV_1 in acute asthma results in improvement of arterial oxygen tension. Hypoxia usually precedes hypercapnia. Rhonchi will not be heard in asthma if air entry is poor. Arterial oxygen tension falls following intravenous aminophylline due to disturbance of pulmonary perfusion. Cyanosis is a poor sign for arterial hypoxaemia as it does not occur until the oxygen saturation has dropped below 75%.

7.3. A B C
Pulmonary oedema in smoke inhalation occurs due to damage of the alveoli, in transfusion reactions due to heart failure and in sea water drowning due to osmosis (sea water is hypertonic, equivalent to 3% saline). In pneumonia there is an exudate. In heart failure due to pulmonary stenosis there is no pulmonary oedema.

7.4. B D E
During an acute asthmatic episode the response to obstruction is recruitment of inspiratory musculature in an attempt to raise lung volume. This results in increased total lung capacity, high negative pleural pressures and increase in functional residual capacity. Because of the high lung volume, compliance is reduced and lung elastic recoil is increased. FEV_1 and tidal volume are decreased.

7.5. Which of the following statements regarding pulmonary function is/are true?

A   Carbon dioxide diffuses more rapidly than oxygen.
B   Compliance is a measure of the elastic characteristic of the respiratory system.
C   Airway resistance is directly related to lung volume.
D   Tidal volume is determined by the functional residual capacity.
E   In normal children, FEV_1 is more than 75% of vital capacity.

7.6. During an episode of acute bronchiolitis

A   lung volume is high.
B   transpulmonary pressure is decreased.
C   alveolar ventilation is initially increased.
D   hypoxia is due to intrapulmonary shunting.
E   gaseous diffusion is the major respiratory physiological disturbance.

7.7. Accepted indications for the removal of adenoids in childhood are

A   mouth breathing.
B   serious postnasal obstruction.
C   nasal escape of air in speech.
D   inspiratory snoring.
E   recurrent otitis media.

7.8. The accepted indications for the removal of tonsils in childhood are

A   peritonsillar abscess.
B   frequent serious upper respiratory tract infections requiring absence from school.
C   eight or more attacks of tonsillitis per year despite chemoprophylaxis.
D   sleep apnoea.
E   recurrent middle ear infections.

7.5. A B E

Carbon dioxide diffusing capacity is 20 times that of oxygen. Compliance expressed as volume/cm of water pressure measures elastic characteristics of the respiratory system. Airway resistance is inversely related to lung volume. Tidal volume is determined by lung compliance and airway resistance. In normal children FEV_1 is more than 75% of total vital capacity.

7.6. A C

In acute bronchiolitis there is recruitment of respiratory muscles in an attempt to hold open the obstructed airways. The respiratory muscle activity leads to extremely negative intrapleural pressures, increased transpulmonary pressures and increased total lung volume. The major physiological disturbance is ventilation–perfusion mismatch. Initial hyperventilation is followed by hypoventilation due to respiratory muscle fatigue. There is no intrapulmonary shunting.

7.7. B

Serious postnasal obstruction due to enlargement of the adenoids is an absolute indication for adenoidectomy. This can be demonstrated by a lateral X-ray of the postnasal space. Mouth-breathing is often due to causes other than enlarged adenoids, e.g. mucosal thickening due to allergy. Nasal escape of air is an absolute contraindication to the removal of adenoid tissue. Unlike expiratory snoring, inspiratory snoring unless related to enlargement of adenoids, is not an indication for adenoidectomy. There is much debate as to whether adenoids should be removed from children who suffer from recurrent middle ear disease; the anatomical linkage of the postnasal space with the middle ear by the Eustachian tube is an enticing argument, but proof by statistical means is lacking.

7.8. B C D

Frequent attacks of real tonsillitis despite appropriate antibacterial prophylaxis is accepted as an indication for tonsillectomy by even the most conservative paediatricians; however, the emphasis is on *real* tonsillitis and not inflamation of the tonsils as part of an upper respiratory tract infection due to viral causes which are not an indication no matter how severe they may be. Peritonsillar abscess was previously regarded as an absolute indication, but effective use of appropriate antibiotic therapy, with surgical drainage where indicated, has produces cures so that in many, perhaps most, cases tonsillectomy is no longer necessary. Sleep apnoea is an absolute indication. There is no association between the tonsils and middle ear infection.

7.9. Tonsillitis due to streptococcal infection can be differentiated from tonsillitis of other aetiology by

A   the presence of exudate on the tonsils.
B   the magnitude of cervical lymph node enlargement.
C   white cell count above 15×10^9/l.
D   the size of the tonsils.
E   none of the above.

7.10. Which of the following statements is/are true of acute otitis media?

A   Fever may be the only presenting feature.
B   Light reflex is altered.
C   Decongestive agents have been demonstrated to be efficacious.
D   Drug of choice for treatment is penicillin.
E   Most infections are bacterial in origin.

7.11. Which of the following statements is/are true about glue ear?

A   More than 30% of all children have seromucus fluid in a middle ear (glue ear) at some time.
B   The prevalence of glue ear drops sharply by mid-primary school age.
C   Ventilating tubes are indicated for children with glue ear having low frequency hearing loss of 30 dB and normal hearing for middle and high frequency.
D   Intermittent hearing loss with head colds in a child with a mild glue ear problem is an indication for inserting ventilating tubes.
E   The amount of scarring of the eardrum depends more on the severity of the middle ear problems than on the frequency of the insertion of ventilating tubes.

7.12. Acute epiglottitis is associated with

A   gradual onset of cough, fever and stridor over several days.
B   infection with parainfluenza virus.
C   *Haemophilus influenzae* type B septicaemia.
D   drooling and difficulty in swallowing.
E   high probability of recurrence.

7.9. E

The only way to distinguish between viral and bacterial tonsillitis is by culture of a throat swab.

7.10. A B

In acute otitis media fever and irritability are the main symptoms, though irritability is not always present. The landmarks of the ear drum are not clear and the light reflex is altered. Decongestive agents are of little use. Most infections are viral in origin. The drug of choice is amoxycillin or trimethoprim with sulphamethoxazole, since secondary bacterial infections are due to *Haemophilus influenzae, Streptococcus pyogenes* or *Streptococcus pneumoniae.*

7.11. A B E

Glue ear of minor severity is often symptomless and has been observed in more than 30% of children at some time. Its prevalence (and the incidence of acute otitis media) drops sharply by mid-primary school age. Low frequency hearing loss of 30 dB is not a significant hearing handicap for children, does not cause irreversible damage and requires no treatment. Provided that there is little handicap at other times, obvious deafness with head colds (which lasts for a few days) is not an indication for ventilating tubes. Tympanic membrane scarring is largely dependent on the severity of middle ear disease.

7.12. C D

The onset of acute epiglottitis is rapid. Respiratory obstruction can occur within hours after the first symptoms of fever and cough. *Haemophilus influenzae* is the causative agent and can be cultured from the blood. The patient has difficulty in swallowing due to the swollen epiglottis, which results in drooling. Recurrence risk is low.

7.13. In laryngomalacia there is characteristically

A   micrognathia.
B   inspiratory stridor.
C   difficulty in feeding.
D   tendency to improvement with age.
E   predisposition to croup.

7.14. Which of the following statements is/are true of acute laryngotracheobronchitis (croup)?

A   Barking cough and hoarse voice are early symptoms.
B   Boys are more likely to be admitted to hospitals than girls.
C   The symptoms frequently respond to salbutamol.
D   The use of nebulized adrenaline is contraindicated.
E   Parainfluenza viruses are the predominant aetiological agents.

7.15. In acute bronchiolitis in a 6-month-old infant

A   the neutrophil count is a good guide to aetiology.
B   oxygen should be used cautiously because of danger of producing hypercapnia.
C   *Haemophilus influenzae* is the most common pathogen.
D   antibiotic treatment has been demonstrated to be effective.
E   respiratory rate and excursion are useful guides to severity of illness.

7.16. Over the period of a day, a 4-month-old infant develops tachypnoea, chest recession, widespread crepitations and expiratory rhonchi. Chest X-ray suggests hyperinflation of the lungs. Which of the following statements is/are correct?

A   Viral studies would show presence of a rhinovirus in more than 25% of cases.
B   The infant has more than a 20% chance of becoming asthmatic later in life.
C   Significant improvement is likely to be obtained by treatment with salbutamol by inhalation.
D   Corticosteroid treatment improves the mortality rate in such cases.
E   The parents may be reassured that the critical period of his illness will not have a duration of more than 48 h.

7.13. B C D E

There is no association between laryngomalacia and micrognathia. The inspiratory stridor is due to partial closure of the larynx during inspiration which results in difficulty with feeding. The symptoms improve with age because the larynx becomes bigger in all directions. Infections result in decreased circumference of the larynx (due to oedema) which manifests as croup.

7.14. A B E

The characteristic features of croup are barking cough and hoarse voice which are worse at night than during the day. The disease appears to be more severe in boys. Parainfluenza viruses are the predominant aetiological agents. It does not respond to treatment with salbutamol by nebulizer though it may respond to administration of adrenaline by nebulizer.

7.15. E

In acute bronchiolitis the neutrophil count is variable. There is no danger in administering oxygen as the condition is of acute onset. Respiratory syncytial virus is the most common causative organism and therefore antibiotics have no effect on the course of the disease. The respiratory rate and excursion indicate the severity of the disease.

7.16. B

The history suggests a diagnosis of bronchiolitis. The rhinoviruses usually cause infections of the nose and rarely cause bronchiolitis. Epidemiological studies have shown that about one-third of patients with a first attack of bronchiolitis develop asthma later in life. Bronchodilators and corticosteroids do not affect the course of the disease. In most cases the disease is most severe for the first 48 h, but death can occur after this period.

7.17. Which of the following statements is/are true of asthma in children?
A   It may present with nocturnal cough without wheeze.
B   It is usually ameliorated by desensitizing injections.
C   If it is exercise-induced it is usually worse after swimming than after running.
D   Exercise-induced asthma can be prevented by salbutamol inhalation prior to exercise.
E   Children are less likely to grow out of it if there is a family history of atopy.

17.18. A foreign body in the respiratory passage can cause
A   atelectasis.
B   unilateral pulmonary hyperinflation.
C   mediastinal displacement.
D   wheezing.
E   recurrent chest infection.

7.19. Which of the following statements is/are true of aspiration of a foreign body?
A   The symptoms associated with aspiration vary with the area of entrapment.
B   A large number of aspirated foreign bodies are foods.
C   The highest risk age group is children aged 4–6 years.
D   Foreign body aspiration should be considered as a possible cause of cough/wheeze in a 2-year-old child even when no history of aspiration is obtained.
E   Foreign bodies are usually radio-opaque.

7.20. In acute bronchopneumonia in a 6-month-old infant
A   the neutrophil count is a good guide to aetiology.
B   oxygen should be used cautiously because of the danger of producing hypercapnoea.
C   *Streptococcus pyogenes* is the commonest pathogen.
D   tetracycline is the most satisfactory antibiotic for initial therapy.
E   respiratory rate and excursion is a useful guide to severity of illness.

7.17. A D E

A reactive airway (asthma) commonly presents with cough at night. Wheezing may not be present. Many agents have been implicated in the aetiology of asthma and therefore desensitization is almost impossible. The main trigger in exercise-induced asthma is dry air, which is less likely to be encountered while swimming. Prior inhalation of salbutamol will prevent exercise-induced asthma by maintaining bronchodilatation. The prognosis for childhood asthma is good, though the asthma is more likely to persist and be severe in those with a family history of atopy.

7.18. A B C D E

The presenting symptoms of foreign body in the respiratory passage depend on whether it causes complete or incomplete obstruction and its location in the respiratory tree. Complete blockage results in atelectasis. Incomplete blockage results in hyperinflation, wheezing and mediastinal displacement to the opposite side. Recurrent chest infection usually occurs with complete blockage.

7.19. A B D

Symptoms of foreign body aspiration include acute apnoea if the foreign body is lodged in the larynx or trachea, severe respiratory distress if the foreign body is lodged in a major bronchus, wheezing when the obstruction is partial, and signs of consolidation when there is superadded infection. Most foreign respiratory bodies are food (and therefore are not radio-opaque) and occur in children below the age of 4 years.

7.20. E

Acute bronchopneumonia is usually due to a bacterial infection. The neutrophil count would suggest such a diagnosis but would not identify the organisms. The most common pathogen is *Haemophilus influenzae*. There is no contraindication for administering oxygen as the condition is of acute onset and there is no danger of respiratory arrest. Tetracycline is not recommended for infants as it stains the teeth. The more severe the disease the more likely the respiratory rate and excursion will be increased, and vice-versa.

7.21. The ultimate outcome in healthy children who survive staphylococcal pneumonia is usually
A   recurrent spontaneous pneumothoraces.
B   chronic respiratory insufficiency.
C   chronic lung abscesses and emphysema.
D   persistent pneumatocoeles.
E   complete resolution.

7.22. A previously well 5-year-old boy presents with a 2-week history of cough, malaise and low grade fever. He has been treated by his local medical officer with amoxycillin with no improvement. Auscultation of his chest reveals widespread crepitations and a chest X-ray shows a generalized interstitial infiltrate. Which of the following statements is/are true?
A   The picture is consistent with viral pneumonitis.
B   The most likely cause is infection with amoxycillin-resistant *Haemophilus influenzae*.
C   Asthma is the likely diagnosis.
D   Positive cold agglutinins will be diagnostic of *Mycoplasma* pneumonitis.
E   The picture is consistent with staphylococcal pneumonia.

7.23. Recurrent respiratory tract infections have significant association with
A   ventricular septal defect.
B   tetralogy of Fallot.
C   gastro-oesophageal reflux.
D   parental smoking.
E   attendance at playschool.

7.24. Which of the following statements is/are true of fibrocystic disease of the pancreas?
A   Intestinal disaccharidase levels are low.
B   Prognosis is unchanged even with optimal management.
C   There is an incidence of 1 in 4 of this condition in the offspring of unaffected siblings.
D   There is an increased incidence of neonatal bowel obstruction.
E   Neonatal screening for immunoreactive trypsin will establish early diagnosis in more than 98% of cases.

7.21. E

In the acute phase, staphylococcal pneumonia could result in recurrent spontaneous pneumothoraces and empyema, lung abscesses and persistent pneumatocoeles. Long-term follow-up will show complete resolution. Chronic respiratory insufficiency is not a feature of staphylococcal pneumonia.

7.22. A

Insiduous onset with persistent symptoms, and widespread changes in the lung with the mildness of the illness suggest a diagnosis of viral pneumonitis rather than a bacterial infection. Clinical history and physical findings are inconsistent with the diagnosis of asthma. While a rise in cold agglutinins titre is suggestive of a diagnosis of *Mycoplasma* pneumonitis, it is not diagnostic.

7.23. A C D E

Recurrent respiratory tract infections occur in ventricular septal defect due to pulmonary congestion, in gastro-oesophageal reflux because of aspiration, and during attendance at playschool because of exposure to other children's infections. Epidemiological studies have shown that parental smoking increases the incidence of recurrent respiratory tract infections. In tetralogy of Fallot there is pulmonary ischaemia and no increased incidence of recurrent respiratory tract infection.

7.24. D

In cystic fibrosis there are no changes in intestinal disaccharidase levels. Over the last 20 years the life expectancy of cystic fibrosis patients has increased from 10 to more than 20 years. The incidence in the offspring of unaffected siblings is approximately 1 in 300 ($1/3 \times 1/4 \times 1/25$). Neonatal bowel obstruction is usually due to meconium ileus or may be due to ileal atresia with or without meconium peritonitis. Neonatal screening with immunoreactive trypsin gives both false positive and false negative results.

7.25. Which of the following statements is/are true of cystic fibrosis?
A   The absence of fat in stools excludes the diagnosis.
B   Heterozygotes can be identified by the sweat test.
C   Males are usually sterile.
D   Intestinal obstruction may be a presenting symptom in the newborn.
E   Life expectancy is less than 20 years.

7.26. In cystic fibrosis
A   the heterozygote frequency is closer to 1 in 25 than 1 in 100.
B   failure to thrive is due to pancreatic insufficiency alone.
C   the high sweat sodium content is of no clinical significance other than for diagnosis.
D   rectal prolapse is a recognized mode of presentation.
E   physiotherapy is an essential component of management.

7.27. In the lung of cystic fibrosis (CF) patients
A   there is a failure of chloride and water secretion into the respiratory mucus layer.
B   there is excessive reabsorption of sodium from the respiratory mucus layer.
C   all chloride channels are CF transmembrane regulator dependent.
D   the transport defect can be overcome by administration of beta-sympathomimetics.
E   the transport defect is most severe in those patients with two delta 508 genes.

7.28. Strategies to overcome the ion transport defect in CF lung include administration of
A   nebulized uridine triphosphate (UTP).
B   nebulized amiloride.
C   oral theophylline.
D   calcium channel blockers.
E   nebulized 6% sodium chloride.

7.25. C D
In cystic fibrosis heterozygotes cannot be identified by the sweat test; males are sterile because of the abnormalities of the vas deferens. It may present with intestinal obstruction due to meconium ileus in the newborn. At present the life expectancy is more than 20 years. Although fat is usually present in the stools, its absence does not exclude the diagnosis.

7.26. A D E
The incidence of cystic fibrosis is 1 in 2500. The heterozygote frequency is 1 in 25. Failure to thrive is due to pancreatic insufficiency and recurrent respiratory tract infections, which require physiotherapy (an essential component of management). The high sweat sodium content can lead to hyponatraemia. Rectal prolapse is a recognized mode of presentation in infancy.

7.27. A B E
In the CF lung the primary transport defect is failure of chloride and water secretion from epithelial cells into the bronchial mucus layer. There is also excessive reabsorption of water and sodium from the mucus layer back into the cell. There are a number of non-CF transmembrane regulator-dependent calcium-activated chloride channels which may be opened using uridine triphosphate. Beta-sympathomimetics have not been shown to overcome the chloride channel defect, which is more severe in homozygous delta 508 patients.

7.28. A B E
Ion transport defect in CF can be modified by nebulized uridine triphosphate, which opens non-CF transmembrane regulator-dependent chloride channels and by amiloride which blocks sodium and water reabsorption. Nebulized 6% sodium chloride replaces both sodium ions and water in mucus secretions. Oral theophylline and calcium channel blockers play no role in the ion transport.

8 Cardiovascular system

8.1. The innocent (physiological) systolic murmur in an 8-year-old child
A   usually changes intensity with posture.
B   is inaudible posteriorly.
C   is maximal in the 4th/5th left interspace.
D   may be associated with a third heart sound.
E   can be musical or high pitched in character.

8.2. The interval between aortic and pulmonary valve closure sounds is increased on inspiration in the normal patient because of
A   descent of the diaphragm.
B   prolongation of left ventricular systole.
C   sinus arrhythmia.
D   prolongation of right ventricular systole.
E   a rise in pulmonary artery pressure.

8.3. A previously well 3-month-old infant presents with reluctance to feed and breathlessness. The pulse rate is 280/min. Which of the following is/are correct?
A   The most likely diagnosis is supraventricular tachycardia (SVT).
B   Diagnosis of Wolff–Parkinson–White (WPW) syndrome can be confirmed during remission by ECG.
C   Facial immersion in ice water is effective treatment.
D   Verapamil is the recommended treatment in this patient.
E   The infant is unlikely to have relapses.

8.4. In which of the following is pulsus paradoxus likely to be present?
A   Pericardial fluid collection due to heart failure.
B   Rheumatic pericarditis.
C   Pneumothorax.
D   Severe asthma.
E   Pericardial fluid collection due to Dressler's syndrome (post-pericardiotomy syndrome).

8.1. A B D E

The innocent systolic murmur is heard in more than 30% of children. It is ejection, musical (frequently sounding like the vibration of a tuning fork), brief in duration, may be attenuated in the sitting position and is intensified by fever, excitement or exercise. It is best heard along the left lower and midsternal border or the pulmonary area and does not radiate to the back, base or apex of the heart.

8.2. D

During inspiration right ventricular ejection time increases due to increased filling of the heart, which increases the interval between the aortic and pulmonary valve closure sounds.

8.3. A B C

The most common cause of heart rates above 220/min at this age is SVT. Rates around 200/min in the neonate may have another cause such as atrial flutter with block or sinus tachycardia. The mechanism is conduction via an accessory pathway. Some patients have WPW syndrome which is apparent on resting ECG in sinus rhythm. Recurrent SVT is a problem in about one-third of these children in the first year of life, and of the two-thirds who do not have early problems about half may have problems in later life. Facial immersion in iced water is frequently effective. As verapamil may cause asystole in the neonate, adenosine is the drug of choice for treatment of resistant cases.

8.4. C D E

Pulsus paradoxus is not a paradox at all. It is an exaggeration of the normal response, i.e. the blood pressure falls with inspiration due to less left-sided filling at that time. This is evident with cardiac compression due to a large pericardial collection or prominent negative intrathoracic pressure during respiration. Unlike Dressler's syndrome, large effusions do not occur in cardiac failure and rheumatic carditis. Asthma and pneumothorax produce large changes in intrathoracic pressure during breathing.

8.5. An otherwise well 3-year-old boy undergoing routine physical examination is repeatedly found to have a blood pressure of 120/90 mmHg when using a cuff covering most of the upper arm. Which of the following is/are appropriate?

A   Take the blood pressure again using a smaller cuff.
B   Examine femoral pulses.
C   Review in 1 year.
D   Measure plasma cholesterol and triglyceride levels.
E   Admit child to hospital urgently.

8.6. Causes of systolic hypertension in children include

A   coarctation of the aorta.
B   complete heart block.
C   acute urinary tract infection.
D   acute glomerulonephritis.
E   neuroblastoma.

8.7. In blood pressure recording

A   the width of the cuff should be two-thirds (or more) of the length of the upper arm.
B   the average pressure in late infancy is approximately 80/55 mmHg by auscultation.
C   the flush pressure approximates to the systolic value.
D   measurement over the lower limbs is more reliable than over the upper limbs.
E   the patient's posture (sitting or supine) has no effect on the measurement.

8.8. Right ventricular hypertrophy in childhood is

A   a characteristic feature of transposition of great vessels.
B   a characteristic feature of tetraology of Fallot.
C   a characteristic feature of tricuspid atresia.
D   diagnosed when the T wave is upright in V1 after 72 h of age.
E   diagnosed when R in V1 exceeds 20 mm.

8.5. B E

The patient has a very high blood pressure which may lead to hypertensive encephalopathy or renal failure. He requires urgent admission and further investigations. The high blood pressure may be due to coarctation of the aorta. Examination of femoral pulses for amplitude and radial–femoral delay as well as measurement of blood pressure in the lower limbs is useful in establishing the diagnosis. A smaller cuff will give an erroneously high blood pressure. There is no indication for measuring serum cholesterol and triglyceride levels.

8.6. A B D E

Coarctation of the aorta and acute glomerulonephritis cause high blood pressure due to disturbance of blood supply to the kidneys. In complete heart block the systolic blood pressure is raised because of increased cardiac output. In neuroblastoma the raised blood pressure is due to catecholamines. Acute urinary tract infection does not cause disturbance in blood pressure.

8.7. A B C

For accurate measurement of blood pressure the width of the cuff should be two-thirds to three-quarters the length of the upper arm. Measurement of blood pressure by the flush method gives approximately the systolic value as blood begins to flow as soon as the cuff's pressure is below the systolic level. The blood pressure at term is 70/50 mmHg. It gradually increases with advancing age reaching a value of 120/75 by the age of 16 years. Blood pressure is affected by posture. Measurement of blood pressure over the lower limbs, though cumbersome, is as reliable as that over the upper limbs.

8.8. A B D E

Right ventricular hypertrophy occurs in transposition of great vessels and tetralogy of Fallot due to increased work-load of the right ventricle. In tricuspid atresia there is left ventricular hypertrophy. The ECG changes of right ventricular hypertrophy include rsR pattern in lead V1, upright T wave in lead V1 after the age of 72 h, and R wave in lead V1 of more than 15 mm.

8.9. Which of the following is/are important in assessing ventricular hypertrophy on electrocardiogram?

A   PR interval.
B   T wave morphology.
C   R wave voltage.
D   Frontal plane axis.
E   Heart rate.

8.10. Which of the following statements is/are correct?

A   Tricuspid atresia is the most common type of cyanotic congenital heart disease.
B   In tetralogy of Fallot the child typically adopts a squatting position after exertion.
C   Notching of the ribs will not be seen in a 6-month-old infant with coarctation of the aorta.
D   The murmur of atrial septal defect is due to flow across the defect.
E   Stridor will resolve in more than 80% of cases by 3 months after surgical correction of vascular ring.

8.11. Which of the following statements is/are true of uncomplicated patent ductus arteriosus in a 2-year-old child?

A   It should be ligated.
B   The patient should be given indomethacin.
C   It may present with cyanosis and clubbing.
D   ECG shows right ventricular hypertrophy.
E   Chest X-ray shows an increase in vascular markings.

8.12. Which of the following is/are true of patent ductus arteriosus (PDA)?

A   The murmur of PDA can be heard in more than 50% of apparently normal babies in the second week of life.
B   If a PDA is present at 6 months of age, the chances of spontaneous closure are less than 3%.
C   A small PDA can be complicated by endoarteritis.
D   Congestive cardiac failure is a recognized complication.
E   Ligation of the PDA should preferably be deferred until the child is older than 4 years.

8.9. B C D

Ventricular hypertrophy is diagnosed by studying the morphology of T waves in the chest leads, voltage of the R waves and the position of the axis of the heart. PR interval indicates the time taken for the electrical impulse to travel from the SA node to the AV node. The heart rate does not reflect the state of the ventricles.

8.10. B C

Tricuspid atresia is an uncommon type of cyanotic heart disease. Transposition of the great vessels is the most common type of cyanotic congenital heart disease at birth. Children with tetralogy of Fallot characteristically assume a squatting position for the relief of dyspnoea due to physical effort but are able to resume physical activity within a few minutes. Notching of the ribs is seen with coarctation of the aorta in later childhood. The murmur of atrial septal defect is due to increased flow of blood across the pulmonary outflow tract and valve. The stridor associated with vascular ring persists after correction in more than 50% of the cases as they have concomitant tracheomalacia.

8.11. A E

Ductus arteriosus which does not close by the age of 2 years needs to be ligated as there is a risk of subacute bacterial endoarteritis and pulmonary hypertension. In patent ductus arteriosus there is increase in pulmonary blood flow which shows as increase in vascular markings on chest X-ray. Right ventricular hypertrophy, cyanosis and clubbing can occur if the patient develops pulmonary hypertension. In uncomplicated patent ductus arteriosus the ECG shows left ventricular hypertrophy.

8.12. B C D

Physiological closure of the ductus arteriosus occurs within 24 h of birth in more than 90% of cases and therefore no murmurs are heard. When the ductus arteriosus persists beyond the neonatal period it is due to structural abnormality (deficiency of both the endothelial and muscular layers) which prevents spontaneous closure. Treatment is best carried out between 1 and 2 years of age (spontaneous closure is uncommon after this age) because of the risk of subacute bacterial endoarteritis, pulmonary hypertension and congestive cardiac failure.

8.13. Which of the following statements is/are true of coarctation of aorta?
A   Hypertension may be the presenting symptom.
B   The left ventricle is frequently hypertrophied
C   A murmur is usually present.
D   The femoral pulse may be of normal amplitude
E   Subacute bacterial endoarteritis prophylaxis should be continued life long after repair.

8.14. Which of the following are classically found in severe aortic stenosis?
A   Small carotid pulse.
B   Fourth heart sound.
C   Prominent left ventricular impulse.
D   Giant A waves
E   Radial–femoral delay.

8.15. Which of the following are found in atrial septal defect?
A   A mid-systolic murmur in the pulmonary area.
B   Fixed splitting of the second heart sound.
C   A systolic thrill.
D   Splitting of the first heart sound.
E   A mid-diastolic murmur at the left lower sternal border.

8.16. Which of the following statements is/are true of atrial septal (septum secundum) defect?
A   The systolic murmur is usually present at birth.
B   The systolic murmur is due to increased flow across pulmonary outflow tract and valve.
C   There is fixed splitting of the second heart sound.
D   The lung fields are plethoric.
E   There is no risk of pulmonary hypertension.

8.13. A B C D E

In coarctation of the aorta, hypertension results from abnormal renal perfusion pressure and wave forms; as a result, the left ventricle is often hypertrophied. The femoral pulse may be normal in the newborn with a large patent ductus arteriosus. In the older patient a fair volume femoral pulse may result from collaterals although it will be delayed. There is usually a murmur (especially after the neonatal age) which is heard best posteriorly. In the older age group collateral noises can also be heard. Lifetime antibiotic prophylaxis is required for treated and untreated coarctation.

8.14. A B C

In severe aortic stenosis the pulse amplitude is low and there is left ventricular enlargement. A prominent fourth heart sound is audible. There is no difference between the radial and femoral pulses and the jugular venous pulse is normal.

8.15. A B E

In atrial septal defect there is an ejection systolic murmur in the pulmonary area due to increased flow across the right ventricular outflow tract, fixed splitting of the second heart sound which is due to constantly increased right ventricular diastolic volume, and prolonged ejection time. There is a mid-diastolic murmur at the lower left sternal border due to high blood flow across the tricuspid valve. There are no thrills and the first heart sound is normal.

8.16. B C D

The murmur of atrial septal defect is not present at birth. It is due to increased flow across the pulmonary outflow tract and valve. The fixed splitting is due to constantly increased right ventricular diastolic volume and prolonged ejection time. The increased blood flow to the lungs is seen as pulmonary plethora on X-ray . Pulmonary hypertension can result from the increased blood flow to the lung.

8.17. Which of the following statements is/are true regarding ventricular septal defects (VSD)?

A All children with large isolated VSD have pulmonary hypertension.

B Pulmonary hypertension is a contraindication to surgical closure of VSD.

C Children with Down syndrome are more likely to develop early pulmonary vascular disease than children with normal chromosomes.

D The presence of mid-diastolic murmur indicates stenosis of the mitral valve.

E The complications are partly dependent on the position of the VSD in the septum.

8.18. Which of the following is/are associated with Fallot's tetralogy?

A Cerebral haemorrhage.

B Squatting.

C Cyanotic spells.

D Cerebral abscess.

E Unsplit second heart sound.

8.19. Which of the following is/are found in children with tetralogy of Fallot?

A The heart appears enlarged on chest X-ray.

B Cyanosis is invariably present by the first birthday.

C Pulmonary valve stenosis must be present to make the diagnosis.

D A right aortic arch is present in more than 15% of cases.

E The aortic valve is smaller than usual.

8.17. A C E

A large VSD does not restrict blood flow between the ventricles, and right ventricle and pulmonary artery pressures will, therefore, be elevated. The presence of pulmonary hypertension needs to be assessed in relation to the pulmonary blood flow. If there is high flow and resistance is low, surgical closure of VSD is possible. Contraindications to repair include high resistance, not pressure in isolation. Children with Down syndrome are more likely to develop high pulmonary resistance at an earlier age, due partly to hypercarbia and partly to pulmonary arterial hypoplasia. The mid-diastolic murmur is due to increased flow across a normal mitral valve. Unlike muscular defects, most doubly committed sub-arterial defects and some peri-membranous defects can cause aortic valve distortion and incompetence.

8.18. B C D E

Cyanotic spells are a particular problem in tetralogy of Fallot during the first 2 years of life. They are associated with a reduction of an already compromised pulmonary blood flow. The second heart sound is single; it is produced by closure of the aortic valve alone since the pulmonary valve closure is not heard. Affected children characteristically assume a squatting position for the relief of breathlessness due to physical effort and the child is usually able to resume physical activity within a few minutes. Cerebral complications such as thrombosis, ischaemia and abscess are recognized complications of tetralogy of Fallot.

8.19. D

Despite the right ventricular hypertrophy, the heart appears normal in size on X-ray due to a small pulmonary artery segment (boot-shaped heart). Many children with tetralogy are born pink and the cyanosis may not be apparent for some years. The pulmonary outflow obstruction is characteristically sub-valvular, and some obstruction at this site is necessary to make the diagnosis. Pulmonary valve abnormalities are the rule but there is not always pulmonary valve stenosis. About 20–25% of cases will have a right aortic arch. The aortic valve is characteristically larger than usual.

8.20. Which of the following statements is/are true of transposition of great arteries?

A   The aorta lies posterior to the pulmonary artery.

B   The aorta receives blood from the left ventricle.

C   Cyanosis usually disappears when 100% oxygen is inspired for 10 min.

D   If a large patent ductus arteriosus is discovered at cardiac catheterization, urgent arrangements for ligation of the duct must be made.

E   Confirmation of diagnosis is urgent.

8.21. Which of the following congenital cardiac defects frequently present with cyanosis?

A   Complete transposition of the great arteries.

B   Tricuspid atresia.

C   Isolated ventricular septal defect.

D   Aortic stenosis.

E   Total anomalous pulmonary venous drainage.

8.22. In congenital heart disease, cyanosis

A   is distinguished from that of respiratory origin by its failure to diminish on breathing 100% oxygen for 10 min.

B   requires at least 5 g/100 ml of reduced Hb for recognition.

C   causes polycythaemia.

D   characteristically causes hyperventilation and respiratory alkalosis.

E   requires urgent investigation.

8.23. Which of the following are associated with finger clubbing?

A   Aortic coarctation.

B   Tricuspid atresia.

C   Tetralogy of Fallot.

D   Asthma.

E   Partial atrioventricular septal defect.

8.20. E

In transposition the aorta lies anterior and to the right of the pulmonary trunk. It receives blood from the right ventricle. Administration of oxygen does not affect the cyanosis. It is important that the ductus arteriosus remains open as it may be the only communication between the heart and the lungs. Immediate investigation by echocardiogram (and treatment by balloon septostomy) are necessary in order to ensure that blood supply to the lungs is maintained (or adequate mixing of venous and arterial blood is possible). Prostaglandins are indicated if there are signs of closure of the ductus arteriosus before investigations can be undertaken.

8.21. A B E

Cyanosis is a presenting symptom of transposition of the great arteries, tricuspid atresia and total anomalous pulmonary venous drainage. In all these conditions there is mixing of arterial with venous blood, which is not the case with aortic stenosis and ventricular septal defect.

8.22. A B C E

Cyanosis of respiratory origin improves following administration of oxygen whereas that due to cardiac disease remains unchanged. Cyanosis is due to the presence of unoxygenated haemoglobin and a minimum of 5 g/100 ml of deoxygenated haemoglobin is necessary for the naked eye to recognized cyanosis. Cyanosis indicates hypoxia, which causes bone marrow hyperplasia resulting in polycythaemia. Patients with cyanotic congenital heart disease need urgent investigation (and treatment) as they may depend on the ductus arteriosus (which may close) to maintain adequate oxygenation. Cyanosis in congenital heart disease does not cause hyperventilation unless complicated by metabolic acidosis.

8.23. B C

Clubbing of fingers occurs in cyanotic congenital heart disease (tricuspid atresia, tetralogy of Fallot), suppurative lung disease (bronchiectasis, cystic fibrosis) and liver disease. It may also be congenital.

8.24. Which of the following statements is/are true of acute rheumatic fever?

A Acute rheumatic carditis with heart failure is a generally accepted indication for corticosteroid treatment.

B Mitral stenosis is a major manifestation of acute rheumatic fever.

C The murmur of aortic incompetence is a recognized feature of acute rheumatic carditis.

D Mitral incompetence occurring during acute rheumatic carditis is permanent unless surgically corrected.

E A transient mid-diastolic murmur is characteristic of acute rheumatic carditis.

8.25. Which of the following statements is/are true of acute rheumatic fever?

A Initial treatment should include penicillin.

B Fever, polyarthralgia and an elevated ASO titre are sufficient to establish the diagnosis.

C The heart murmur most often heard in acute rheumatic carditis is the murmur of mitral incompetence.

D Rheumatic chorea has a special tendency to occur as an isolated symptom in an otherwise well person.

E After acute rheumatic carditis, prophylaxis with oral penicillin is recommended.

8.26. Prophylaxis with penicillin against subacute bacterial endocarditis in a patient with congenital heart disease is

A inadequate treatment for a child requiring abdominal surgery.

B not necessary in a patient with a very small ventricular septal defect.

C adequate treatment in a patient requiring dental treatment.

D not indicated in a patient who has had his ductus arteriosus ligated and who has no other cardiac lesions.

E indicated if the patient has an upper respiratory tract infection.

8.24. A C E

Acute rheumatic fever can result in pancarditis. The mitral and aortic valves are most commonly involved. In the acute phase, involvement of the mitral valve is manifested as a mid-diastolic murmur which may resolve. Mitral stenosis is a late complication of involvement of the valve. Lesions of the aortic valve result in aortic incompetence or, less commonly, aortic stenosis. Mitral incompetence in the acute phase may resolve spontaneously. Carditis with cardiac enlargement and/or heart failure is an indication for corticosteroid therapy.

8.25. A C E

The diagnosis of acute rheumatic fever is based on Jones', criteria which include two major manifestations (carditis, polyarthritis, chorea, erythema marginatum, subcutaneous nodules) or one major and two minor manifestations (fever, arthralgia, previous rheumatic fever or rheumatic heart disease, raised ASO titre, raised ESR, leucocytosis, C-reactive protein, prolonged P-R interval). The mitral valve is most commonly involved, and this usually presents with the murmur of mitral incompetence. As the relationship between acute rheumatic carditis and streptococcal infection is well established, appropriate treatment consists of therapeutic dosages of penicillin followed by long-term penicillin prophylaxis. Rheumatic chorea is often accompanied by emotional lability, deterioration in school performance and poor coordination. The affected muscles are weak and the deep tendon reflexes are variable.

8.26. A C D

For abdominal surgery, prophylaxis against subacute bacterial endocarditis requires gentamicin (for Gram-negative organisms of gut) in addition to penicillin; this should be offered to all patients with congenital or acquired heart disease. Penicillin is adquate treatment for the patient requiring dental treatment. It is not indicated for a patient who had his ductus arteriosus ligated and who has an upper respiratory tract infection.

8.27. A 1-year-old boy is referred for evaluation of a convulsion. He is found to have cardiomegaly, a pulse rate of 45/min, a 2/6 systolic murmur at the base and a 1-2/6 diastolic murmur at the left lower sternum edge and apex. Which of the following statements is/are true?

A   This patient probably has structural heart anomalies.
B   The patient's mother is likely to have autoantibodies.
C   This patient needs a pacemaker.
D   The pulse pressure is likely to be increased.
E   Many patients with this condition can lead a normal active life without treatment.

8.28. Which of the following statements is/are true regarding Williams' syndrome?

A   Supravulvar aortic stenosis is usually progressive.
B   Peripheral pulmonary artery stenosis is a well-recognized association.
C   Distal arch anomalies are more common than in the general population.
D   Neonates and infants are irritable and pcor feeders.
E   It is autosomal recessive.

8.27. B C D E

The history suggests a diagnosis of congenital heart block. This is usually due to maternal autoantibodies, though it is occasionally a result of congenitally corrected transposition with ventricular inversion or other anomalies. The presence of systolic and diastolic murmurs, cardiomegaly and wide pulse pressure are due to increased stroke volume rather than structural cardiac anomalies. Although most children do not need pacemakers at this age, this infant needs prompt insertion of a pacemaker as the resting heart rate is only 45 and there has been a convulsion. Unless there are syncopes, most patients lead a normal active life.

8.28. A B C D

Supra-aortic stenosis is the most common lesion in Williams' syndrome and is usually progressive. Many children have peripheral pulmonary artery stenosis which may improve with time. Distal arch hypoplasia (not necessarily coarctation) is not infrequent. These infants are extremely irritable and difficult to feed in the neonatal period. The 'cocktail party' personality does not develop until a few years later. Genetic studies suggest that when the anomaly is familial it is transmitted as an autosomal dominant trait with variable expression.

9 Haematology and oncology

9.1. You are asked to see a 5-week-old baby whose birth weight was 1.3603 kg. Delivery was normal and his haemoglobin at birth was normal. The baby has fed and gained weight well. However, his haemoglobin is now 8 g/100 ml. You would expect the anaemia to be due to
A   increase in blood volume.
B   lack of iron in the diet.
C   normal attrition and non-replacement of red blood cells.
D   increased fragility of red cells.
E   lack of iron absorption.

9.2. Which of the following haematological value/s is/are within normal limits?
A   Haemoglobin of 14 g/100 ml in a 1-month-old boy.
B   White cell count of $12 \times 10^9/l$ with 16% neutrophils in a 6-month-old boy.
C   White cell count of $15 \times 10^9/l$ with 70% lymphocytes in a 6-month-old boy.
D   Haemoglobin F of 2% in a 1-year-old boy.
E   Platelet count of $80 \times 10^9/l$ in a normal full-term infant.

9.3. Fetal haemoglobin
A   has a higher iron content than adult haemoglobin.
B   has higher oxygen binding capacity.
C   is the sole haemoglobin that can be identified during fetal life.
D   forms the major fraction of total haemoglobin during late infancy.
E   is resistant to alkali denaturation.

9.4. Causes of iron deficiency in a 2-year-old child include
A   consumption of more than 1 litre of milk a day.
B   feeding fads.
C   acute glomerulonephritis.
D   coeliac disease.
E   premature birth.

9.1. A C
Premature infants grow very rapidly and increase their blood volume. The bone marrow is unable to produce enough red blood cells to maintain the haemoglobin. Anaemia in premature infants also occurs because of 'physiological hypoplasia' of the marrow. Iron deficiency anaemia of prematurity does not appear until the age of 3–6 months. Although the blood of premature infants may contain larger amounts of fetal haemoglobin, which may cause slightly increased fragility of the red cells, it does not account for the anaemia. Absorption of iron is normal compared with full-term infants.

9.2. A B C D
The values mentioned in A, B, C and D are normal. Normal platelet counts in a full-term infant are $150–400 \times 10^9/l$.

9.3. B E
Fetal haemoglobin has the same iron content as adult haemoglobin but has greater affinity for oxygen, which shifts the oxygen dissociation curve to the left. Although it is the major form of haemoglobin in fetal life (90% at 28 weeks, 70% at term), the proportion of adult haemoglobin progressively increases as gestation progresses and very small amounts (less than 2%) of haemoglobin F are present in late infancy. It is resistant to alkali denaturation.

9.4. A B D
Iron deficiency occurs in children consuming large quantities of milk (which is poor in iron content) as they do not take other foods because their caloric needs are met by the milk intake. In acute glomerulonephritis the blood loss in the urine is very small and therefore iron deficiency does not occur. Iron deficiency anaemia in premature infants usually occurs between 3 and 6 months of age. Iron deficiency may result from feeding fads because such foods may not contain iron; in coeliac disease iron deficiency may be a consequence of poor absorption of iron.

9.5. Which of the following anaemias is/are associated with hypochromic red cells?
A Lead poisoning.
B Sideroblastic anaemia.
C Thalassaemia minor.
D Pulmonary haemosiderosis.
E Acute blood loss.

9.6. An 11-month-old child with parents of Greek origin presents with irritability and pallor. He has a haemoglobin level of 7 g/100 ml and hypochromic microcytic blood film. His serum ferritin level is below normal. Which of the following statements is/are correct?
A He probably has beta-thalassaemia ma_or.
B A dietary history is important.
C Occult bleeding should be excluded.
D The parents should be tested for evidence of thalassaemia trait if this has not been done before.
E A low serum ferritin indicates depletion of iron stores.

9.7. An 11-month-old boy presents with pallor. There is no bruising or hepatosplenomegaly. His mother is of Italiaa and his father is of English origin. His haemoglobin is 3.5 g/100 ml. The blood film shows hypochromic microcytic red cells and the white cells show normal morphology. Which of the following is/are correct?
A This disease is a sex-linked disorder.
B A dietary history is very important.
C Long-term treatment with blood transfusion will be required.
D A bone marrow examination is indicated.
E Adequate intake of cereals might have prevented this child's anaemia.

9.5. A B C D

The hypochromic, microcytic anaemias are now referred to as the microcytic anaemias because automated machines measure blood cell size and not the haemoglobin content. Lead poisoning affects delta aminolevulinic acid metabolism and thus haem production. Sideroblastic anaemia may be idiopathic or due to disorders of haem metabolism. Thalassaemia minor is associated with a decrease in globin. Pulmonary haemosiderosis leads to iron deficiency anaemia due to chronic loss of blood into the lung. In acute blood loss the anaemia is normocytic or macrocytic.

9.6. B C D E

In the presence of hypochromic microcytic anaemia and low serum ferritin levels the diagnosis is iron deficiency anaemia. A peripheral blood film will show nucleated red blood cells and target cells in patients with thalassaemia. Poor iron intake (no solids in the diet) and occult blood loss are the most common causes of iron deficiency in infants and children. In view of the ethnic background, it is important to ensure that the parents do not have thalassaemia trait. Serum ferritin is the most reliable blood test that allows the evaluation of iron reserves.

9.7. B E

Hypochromic microcytic anaemia occurs due to iron deficiency. There may be slight splenomegaly and hepatomegaly, unlike thalassaemia major in which the liver and spleen are much enlarged, and there are target cells and nucleated red blood cells. In an 11-month-old child the most likely cause of iron deficiency is a diet deficient in iron (no solids in the diet). Cereals are a very rich source of iron as some of them are fortified with iron. The infant can be treated with supplemental iron and blood transfusions are not indicated. Leukaemia is an unlikely diagnosis because the morphology of the white cells is normal. The parents' ethnic origins are not relevant in iron deficiency anaemia.

9.8. Megaloblastic anaemia is likely to occur in infants
A   fed on soya formula.
B   fed on goats' milk.
C   undergoing resection of ileum.
D   with gastro-oesophageal reflux.
E   with colostomy for Hirschsprung's disease.

9.9. Which of the following is/are features of haemolytic anaemias?
A   Reticulocytosis.
B   Raised haptoglobin.
C   Raised conjugated bilirubin.
D   Hypochromic erythrocytes.
E   Urobilin in urine.

9.10. Which of the following statements is/are true of β thalassaemia major?
A   There is a defect in synthesis of haemoglobin A.
B   The condition may be readily recognizable in the newborn by haemoglobin electrophoresis.
C   Abnormalities will usually be found in the blood film of both parents.
D   Spherocytes are characteristically found in the peripheral blood film.
E   It can be diagnosed *in utero* by amniotic fluid examination.

9.11. Which of the following is/are true of β thalassaemia major?
A   The infant is anaemic at birth.
B   Fetal haemoglobin levels are elevated at the time of diagnosis.
C   The likelihood of a sibling being similarly affected is 1 in 2.
D   Parents are likely to have raised levels of fetal haemoglobin exceeding 20%.
E   Desferrioxamine should not be administered until after the age of 6 years because of toxic effects.

9.8. B C

Megaloblastic anaemia in infants fed on goats' milk is due to deficiency of folic acid. That due to resection of ileum is due to vitamin B_{12} malabsorption. Anaemia due to gastro-oesophageal reflux is due to blood loss leading to iron deficiency. There is no anaemia associated with soya formula or Hirschsprung's disease.

9.9. A E

In haemolytic anaemias, the reticulocyte count is increased, haptoglobin levels are decreased, red blood cells are normochromic and unconjugated bilirubin levels are increased. There is increased urobilin but no bile in the urine.

9.10. A C

In thalassaemia major there is impaired synthesis of beta chains of haemoglobin which are required for the synthesis of haemoglobin A. As a result haemoglobin F is formed. As haemoglobin F is normally present in the newborn period, haemoglobin electrophoresis will not establish the diagnosis. Blood of the parents (heterozygotes) contains elevated levels of haemoglobin A_2 (3.5–7%) and haemoglobin F (2–6%). Some heterozygotes may have normal levels of HbA_2 with raised levels of HbF (5–15%) only.

9.11. B

Thalassemia major is diagnosed by demonstration of raised levels of fetal haemoglobin, which is normally present in the newborn infant. The disease is autosomal recessive, and the incidence in siblings is, therefore, 1 in 4. Haemoglobin F levels in heterozygotes (parents) are usually less than 5% though in some cases may be up to 15%. Haemoglobin A_2 levels vary between 3.5 and 7%. Desferrioxamine could be administered at any age, although it is usually not commenced before the age of 1 year because of technical problems. The infant is not anaemic at birth.

9.12. Which of the following statements is/are true of hereditary spherocytosis (HS)?

A About 50% of affected infants have moderately severe neonatal jaundice.
B The presence of spherocytes on examination of a blood film in the new-born confirms the diagnosis.
C Aplastic crises occur due to parvovirus infection.
D Intravascular haemolysis is a common feature.
E Red blood cell osmotic fragility is increased.

9.13. Which of the following is/are true of hereditary spherocytosis?

A It is inherited as an autosomal dominant.
B The symptoms are relieved by splenectomy.
C Pigment gallstones occur in over 20% of children before the age of 14 years.
D Patients with this condition should avoid oxidizing agents such as primaquin.
E The red cell morphology reverts to normal after splenectomy.

9.14. A 4-year-old boy presents with anaemia and dark urine. Urine examination is positive for blood but no red blood cells are seen on microscopy. Which of the following statements is/are correct?

A Recent dietary history is important.
B A raised blood pressure would suggest a diagnosis of acute nephritis.
C The most likely diagnosis is haemolytic–uraemic syndrome.
D The condition is unlikely to be life threatening.
E The family history of jaundice is important in elucidating the diagnosis.

9.15. Rh-immune globulin prevents Rh isoimmunization by

A neutralizing Rh-immune globulin formed by the Rh-negative mother.
B coating Rh-positive cells and preventing exposure of the Rh antigen to the maternal immune mechanism.
C stimulating the mother to produce anti-Rh human globulin which destroys actively produced Rh antibody.
D competing with Rh antigen for albumin binding sites.
E eliminating Rh-positive cells from the maternal circulation.

9.12. A C E
About half of all newborn infants with hereditary spherocytosis develop jaundice severe enough to require phototherapy. In the newborn period ABO incompatibility can present with spherocytes in the peripheral blood film; this can be confused with hereditary spherocytosis. Aplastic crises occur with parvovirus infections. There is usually haemolysis and decreased red cell production rather than true aplasia. There is no intravascular haemolysis. Red cell osmotic fragility is increased because the red blood cell is spherical instead of biconcave.

9.13. A B
Hereditary spherocytosis is autosomal dominant. As the majority of cells are destroyed by the spleen, splenectomy relieves the symptoms. Although gall-stones have been reported in children as young as 4–5 years of age, in most cases they occur in late childhood or adolescence. Haemolysis occurs because of the abnormality of the cells and not due to oxidizing agents. Red cell morphology remains unchanged after splenectomy.

9.14. A D E
The history suggests intravascular haemolysis with haemoglobinuria. Severe haemolysis occurs in G-6-PD deficiency on ingestion of fava beans. A family history of jaundice indicates the presence of a familial haemolytic anaemia. In acute nephritis and haemolytic–uraemic syndrome red blood cells are seen on microscopy. Though the anaemia may be severe, the haemolysis is self limiting.

9.15. E
Rh-immune globulin eliminates Rh-positive cells from the maternal circulation thereby preventing the mother from being isoimmunized. The Rh-immune globulin formed by the Rh-negative mother is the same as the administered Rh-immune globulin and therefore it cannot neutralize it or stimulate the production of anti-Rh immune globulin. The Rh antigen does not bind to albumin to produce antibodies. The Rh-immune globulin does not just coat the Rh-positive cells but actively destroys them, thus eliminating them from the maternal circulation.

9.16. An infant or young child whose spleen is removed following traumatic rupture has an increased risk of developing

A thrombocytopenia.
B haemolytic anaemia.
C leukaemia.
D polycythemia.
E severe bacterial infection.

9.17. A preponderance of lymphocytes in the differential white cell count is found in

A infants at birth.
B infants at 3 months.
C children aged 10 years.
D whooping cough.
E infectious mononucleosis.

9.18. Idiopathic thrombocytopenic purpura in children

A often follows a viral infection.
B typically has a chronic course, with relapses following each remission.
C is characteristically associated with moderate splenomegaly.
D is associated with a reduction of megakaryocytes on bone marrow examination.
E requires splenectomy in more than 20% of cases.

9.19. Platelet transfusion may be indicated in patients with

A haemophilia.
B Henoch–Schönlein purpura.
C aplastic anaemia.
D chronic idiopathic thrombocytopenic purpura.
E lupus erythematosus.

9.16. E

Removal of the spleen alters host resistance and increases the risk of life threatening infection by meningococci, pneumococci and *H. influenzae* (septicaemia or meningitis). Immediately after splenectomy platelet levels are increased; they may be normal later. There is no increased risk of haemolytic anaemia, leukaemia or polycythemia.

9.17. B D E

At birth infants have a lower lymphocyte count. After the first week of life they have relative lymphocytosis before adult proportions are approached at the age of 10 years. There is lymphocytosis in whooping cough and infectious mononucleosis. In the latter condition the lymphocytes are atypical.

9.18. A

Approximately 60% of patients with idiopathic thrombocytopenic purpura give a history of preceding viral infections. Relapses rarely follow a remission. There is no splenomegaly and megakaryocytes are either normal or increased. About 90% of children regain normal platelet counts within 9–12 months of onset of disease.

9.19. C

Bleeding in haemophilia is due to factor VIII or factor IX deficiency. In Henoch–Schönlein purpura it is due to vascular fragility. Platelet transfusion is indicated in bleeding episodes of aplastic anaemia. It is not indicated in chronic idiopathic thrombocytopenic purpura because bleeding episodes are extremely rare. In immune thrombocytopenic purpura due to lupus erythematosus transfused platelets are rapidly destroyed and are of little benefit to the patient.

9.20. A boy aged 6 years has a history of severe bruising and petechiae of several days' duration. He is not anaemic. There is no enlargement of liver or spleen. Which of the following statements is/are true of this patient?

A The most likely diagnosis is idiopathic thrombocytopenic purpura.

B Bone marrow examination will show numerous megakaryocytes.

C Complete recovery would be expected in 3–8 weeks in more than 70% of cases.

D Bleeding in joints is a likely complication.

E Splenectomy is recommended if the disease is still active after 3–4 months.

9.21. Which of the following statements is/are true of anaphylactoid (Henoch–Schönlein) purpura?

A The platelet count is less than $100 \times 10^9/l$.

B Microscopic haematuria may persist for more than 1 year.

C Intussusception is a recognized complication.

D The arthritis may lead to joint deformity.

E There is evidence to suggest that it is an immune complex disease.

9.22. Haemophilia A is associated with

A petechiae.

B prolonged skin bleeding time (BT).

C prolonged prothrombin time (PT).

D prolonged activated partial thromboplastin time (APTT)

E haemarthrosis.

9.23. A 5-year-old child receiving maintenance chemotherapy for acute lymphoblastic leukaemia presents with a temperature of 39°C, but no other symptoms. Appropriate immediate measures include

A full blood count.

B blood culture.

C bone marrow aspiration.

D checking respiratory rate.

E lumbar puncture.

9.20. A B C

A tendency to bruising and petecheal haemorrhages support the diagnosis of idiopathic thrombocytopenic purpura, in which there are numerous megakaryocytes in the bone marrow. The majority of these patients recover in 6 weeks. There is no bleeding in the joints as the other clotting factors are normal. Splenectomy is indicated only if the disease is severe and fails to respond to corticosteroids and gammaglobulins or if chronic (more than one year).

9.21. B C E

Henoch–Schönlein purpura is the most common form of systemic vasculitis in children, and is presumed to be an immune complex disease since immunofluorescence shows mesangial deposits of IgA in association with IgG, C3 and fibrin. The platelet count is normal. The principal manifestations are arthritis or arthralgia which causes no deformity, abdominal pain sometimes accompanied by intussusception, urticarial/purpuric rash involving the buttocks and lower limbs and haematuria, which may persist for years. The renal lesion sometimes progresses to chronic renal failure.

9.22. D E

Haemophilia A is caused by factor VIII deficiency. It results in haemarthrosis because of bleeding in the joints which fails to stop. As the platelets are normal, there is no increase in petechiae or bleeding time. Prothombin time is normal. There is prolonged APTT which is corrected by addition of plasma but not of serum.

9.23. A B D

Leukaemic children receiving chemotherapy who develop fever are most likely to have septicaemia or respiratory infections. Diagnosis is made by full blood count which shows leucopenia, blood culture and counting the respiratory rate (chest signs are rarely present). Meningitis is extremely rare and bone marrow aspiration is not indicated.

9.24. A parent of an 8-year-old child receiving chemotherapy for leukaemia is notified from school that another child has chickenpox. Which of the following is/are necessary in the management of this child?

A   Establish whether the leukaemic child has had chickenpox.
B   Give a course of acyclovir.
C   Establish the proximity of contact in school.
D   Establish the timing of contact in school.
E   Give a pooled gammaglobulin injection.

9.25. Which of the following is/are true about the toxic effects of anticancer drugs?

A   Cyclophosphamide may cause cystitis.
B   Vincristine causes myopathy.
C   Corticosteroids cause a peripheral neuropathy.
D   Anthracyclines may be cardiotoxic.
E   Methotrexate causes gastrointestinal ulceration.

9.26. Acute lymphoblastic leukaemia

A   is the most common childhood malignancy.
B   is accompanied by splenomegaly in more than half of newly diagnosed children.
C   is excluded if no blast cells are seen in the peripheral blood film.
D   seldom produces intracranial complications.
E   treatment places the the child at grave risk from infection by varicella and measles.

9.27. Enlarged lymph nodes on the lateral side of the neck are more likely to be malignant if

A   they are painful and tender.
B   they are bigger than 2 cm.
C   they are discrete and firm.
D   the chest X-ray is normal.
E   the nodes appear very rapidly.

9.24. C D
Chickenpox is a very serious disease in a leukaemic child and past infection does not prevent the child from reinfection. Acylovir has not been shown to be useful prophylactically. It is important to establish the proximity of the contact and to establish the time of contact as it will allow the incubation period to be monitored closely. Pooled gammaglobulin is not useful though hyperimmune gammaglobulin is effective when given within 72 h of exposure.

9.25. A D E
Side effects of cyclophosphamide are haemorrhagic cystitis, colitis, pulmonary interstital fibrosis and cardiomyopathy (when given in large doses). Methotrexate causes gastrointestinal ulceration, skin rashes, central nervous system symptoms (aphasia, hemiparesis, motor neuropathy) and pneumonitis. Anthracyclines (daunorubicin hydrochloride) cause cardiotoxicity and alopecia. Vincristine causes alopecia and peripheral neuropathy but no myopathy. Corticosteroids may cause myopathy but not peripheral neuropathy.

9.26. A B E
Acute lymphoblastic leukaemia is the most common childhood malignancy (intracranial malignancy is second). Splenomegaly is a common finding. Treatment consists of chemotherapy, which lowers the host immune responses and makes them liable to severe infections with varicella and measles. Blast cells are not seen in the peripheral blood in aleukaemic leukaemia. CNS infiltration is present in 5% of children at diagnosis but accounts for 20% of relapses.

9.27. B C
In cervical lymph node malignancy the lymph nodes are painless, firm, discrete and larger than 2 cm. The enlargement is most commonly due to non-Hodgkin's lymphoma or Hodgkin's disease, with acute lymphocytic leukaemia and acute myeloid leukaemia being next common. Chest X-ray may be normal in these conditions. Painful and tender lymph nodes are not a feature of malignancy. The rapidity with which the nodes appear does not distinguish between enlargement due to infection or malignancy.

9.28. In non-Hodgkin's lymphoma in childhood, which of the following statements is/are true?

A   Immunodeficiencies predispose to the development of this form of lymphoma.

B   Radiation therapy is essential for most patients.

C   An abdominal mass is a rare presentation.

D   The bone marrow may be the first site of relapse.

E   Chemotherapy programmes are designed for particular subtypes of disease.

9.29. The differential diagnosis in a 3-year-old child with a palpable right abdominal mass includes

A   Wilms' tumour.

B   non-Hodgkin's lymphoma.

C   mesoblastic nephroma.

D   neuroblastoma.

E   hepatoblastoma.

9.30. A boy aged 4 years has a large abdominal mass. X-ray and CT scan of his chest showed multiple round intrapulmonary metastases. Which of the following is/are likely?

A   Neuroblastoma.

B   Wilms' tumour.

C   Non-Hodgkin's lymphoma.

D   Hodgkin's disease.

E   Rhabdomyosarcoma.

9.31. A 4-year-old child presents with stridor and acute respiratory distress. On examination there is an area of increased dullness across the middle of the anterior chest wall but no other evidence of organomegaly elsewhere. Blood count shows haemoglobin 140 g/l, leucocytes 15×10^9/l (neutrophils 65%, lymphocytes 25%, monocytes 10%), platelets 350×10^9/l. Which of the following procedures should be undertaken within the first 24 h?

A   Bone marrow examination.

B   Biopsy of cervical lymph nodes, even if not enlarged.

C   Chest x-ray.

D   CT or ultrasound of abdomen.

E   Urgent thoracotomy regardless of results of previous investigations.

9.28. A D E
Both congenital and acquired immunodeficiencies predispose to non-Hodgkin's lymphoma. Radiotherapy is rarely used except to treat central nervous system disease. An abdominal mass may be present in 30% of cases. Bone marrow may be involved at diagnosis or may be the first site of relapse. Non-Hodgkin's lymphoma may be of the T or B cell lineage and requires specific and different combinations of drugs.

9.29. A B D E
Wilms' tumour arises from the kidneys, neuroblastoma from the adrenal gland and hepatoblastoma from the liver, all of which can represent as a mass on the right side of the abdomen. Mesoblastic nephroma is a congenital tumour and occurs in children under the age of 2 years. Non-Hodgkin's abdominal lymphomas occur most frequently in the ileocaecal region and present as an abdominal mass, intestinal obstruction or intussusception.

9.30. B E
Wilms' tumour and rhabdomyosarcoma are two malignancies that present with abdominal masses and intrapulmonary metastases. In neuroblastoma the metastases are in the orbit, liver and bone marrow. In Hodgkin's disease and non-Hodgkin's lymphoma the secondary lesions occur simultaneously in many lymph nodes. The lung secondaries in Hodgkin's disease, non-Hodgkin's lymphomas and neuroblastomas are not coin-shaped.

9.31. A C D
The clinical features indicate a mass in the upper mediastinum. At this age the most likely diagnosis is T cell non-Hodgkin's lymphoma. An X-ray of the chest is required to confirm the clinical impression. Bone marrow aspirate is necessary to make the diagnosis since marrow involvement is common and thoracotomy or other invasive procedures should be avoided. CT or ultrasound of abdomen, gallium scan and diagnostic lumbar puncture are important staging procedures.

9.32. Which of the following statements is/are true of Wilms' tumour?

A   It is the most common malignant tumour of the genitourinary tract of childhood.

B   With current treatment 5-year survival exceeds over 60%.

C   There is an increased incidence of congenital hemihypertrophy in this tumour.

D   Prognosis is less favourable in children under 2 years of age.

E   It presents with haematuria in more than 70% of cases.

9.33. Neuroblastoma

A   has a worse prognosis in the first year of life.

B   may be a cause of paraplegia.

C   does not usually respond to cytotoxic drugs.

D   may sometimes be cured by bone marrow transplantation.

E   may be monitored by testing urinary catecholamines.

9.34. Which of the following statements is/are true of neuroblastoma?

A   It commonly presents as an abdominal mass.

B   IVP commonly reveals displacement and compression of the pelvicalyceal pattern.

C   It mainly affects children between 5 and 10 years of age.

D   Metastasis to bone is unusual.

E   A specific aid to preoperative diagnosis is measurement of urinary excretion of catecholamines.

9.35. Which of the following statements about retinoblastoma is/are true?

A   Systemic metastases are usually present at diagnosis.

B   It often presents with leukocoria.

C   It may be bilateral.

D   Some cases are dominantly inherited.

E   It has a 50% overall mortality in Western countries in spite of the best available treatment.

9.32. A B C
Wilms' tumour accounts for almost all renal neoplasms in childhood. It is often accompanied by other congenital anomalies, including genitourinary anomalies (4.4%), hemihypertrophy (2.9%) and sporadic aniridia (1.1%). Prognosis is better in children diagnosed before the age of 2 years and cure rates of more than 60% have been reported in all stages of Wilms' tumour. Microscopic or macroscopic haematuria occurs in 10–25% of cases.

9.33. B D E
The earlier the age of onset of neuroblastoma the better the prognosis. Paraplegia is caused by direct extension of the tumour into the spinal foramina. Treatment of choice is cytotoxic drugs and radiation. In disseminated disease following extensive chemotherapy and radiation therapy, bone marrow transplantation may be curative. The level of urinary catecholamines indicates progression or recurrence of the tumour.

9.34. A B E
Neuroblastoma is one of the most common tumours presenting as an intra-abdominal mass other than Wilms' tumour. The tumour displaces the kidney downwards and thereby distorts the pelvicalyceal pattern. The usual age of presentation is less than 5 years. Metastases to bones and bone marrow are common. Catecholamine excretion in urine is increased and is responsible for hypertension.

9.35. B C D
Retinoblastoma spreads by local extension and reaches subarachnoid space and brain. Haematogenous spread is rare. Leukocoria (a creamy-white pupillary reflex) is the first sign other than strabismus and loss of vision. Forty percent of retinoblastomas are inherited; inheritance may be autosomal dominant. The tumour may appear in the other eye years later. Outcome is good if diagnosed and treated early (90% survival).

9.36. Clinical features of posterior midline cerebellar tumour include

A   visual field defects.
B   truncal ataxia.
C   stiff neck.
D   dystonia.
E   papilloedema.

9.37. Which of the following statements is/are true of brain tumours in childhood?

A   They are a rare form of malignancy.
B   Most tumours are localized below the tentorium.
C   Hemiparesis is a frequent form of presentation.
D   Papilloedema is infrequent.
E   Medulloblastoma is the most common tumour.

9.36. B C E

The classical signs of posterior midline tumours are ataxia, stiff neck and raised intracranial pressure causing papilloedema. There is no visual field defect (unless there is severe papilloedema) or dystonia.

9.37. B E

Next to leukaemias brain tumours are the commonest form of malignancy in childhood. The tumours are most often infratentorial and histologically are medulloblastomas. Raised intracranial pressure causing papilloedema is common and hemiparesis is rare.

10 Nephrology, including fluid and electrolytes

10.1. Which of the following statements is/are correct?

A Glomerular filtration rate (corrected for surface area) is higher in babies than in older children.

B Protein in the urine is diagnostic of urinary tract infection.

C Infants are able to concentrate their urine less effectively than 10-year-old children.

D The urinary protein in nephrotic syndrome is predominantly tubular in origin.

E Significant urinary losses of IgG do not occur in childhood steroid-responsive nephrotic syndrome.

10.2. Which of the following statements regarding glomerular function is/are correct?

A Blood urea level in babies correlates well with glomerular filtration rate.

B Serum creatinine levels usually fall with increasing age.

C Clinical signs and symptoms of renal failure do not manifest until more than 70% of glomerular filtration rate is lost.

D Glomerular filtration rate can be measured by renal clearance rate of ^{99m}Tc DTPA.

E Glomerular filtration rate can be determined from a formula utilizing the child's height and plasma creatinine.

10.3. Which of the following statements about renal tubular function is/are true?

A Glucose is reabsorbed in the proximal renal tubule.

B Most of the sodium reabsorption occurs in the distal renal tubule.

C Most of the potassium excreted in the urine is derived from secretion by distal renal tubule and the collecting duct.

D Reabsorption of phosphate is inhibited by parathyroid hormone.

E Urine acidification is carried out in the distal renal tubule.

10.1. C E
The rate of glomerular filtration increases until growth ceases towards the end of the second decade of life. Urinary tract infection can only be diagnosed by demonstrating a high colony count in a properly collected specimen of urine. Maximal urinary concentrating capacity of a well newborn infant is 600–700 mosmol/kg water; this increases progressively to 1000 mosmol/kg in older children and adults. The urinary protein loss in nephrotic syndrome is mainly glomerular. Unlike albumin, gammaglobulins are large molecules and are not lost in urine in children with nephrotic syndrome.

10.2. C D E
Blood urea in babies can be increased by increased protein intake. Serum creatinine levels rise with increasing age. Glomerular filtration rate is very low before signs and symptoms of renal failure appear. It can be measured by renal clearance rate of ^{99m}Tc DTPA and can be calculated from the child's height and plasma creatinine.

10.3. A C D E
Glucose and amino acids are reabsorbed in the proximal tubule in conjunction with sodium transport. About 60% of the filtered sodium is isotonically reabsorbed in the proximal tubule, 25% in the ascending limb of the loop of Henle in association with the active transport of chloride and the remainder in the distal tubule and collecting duct. The latter is mediated in part by aldosterone. Sodium excretion is closely related to the extracellular fluid volume and may be modified by factors that regulate the extracellular fluid volume. Almost all the potassium excreted in the urine is derived from secretion by distal tubule and the collecting ducts. Phosphate is reabsorbed in the proximal tubule and its reabsorption is inhibited by parathyroid hormone. Urine acidification occurs in the distal renal tubule by hydrogen ion secretion, which is in part mineralocorticoid dependent and partly due to production of ammonia.

10.4. A previously well 1-year-old girl presents with fever (temperature 38.7°C) and irritability of 24 h duration. Physical examination is essentially normal with no obvious source of fever identified. The labia are cleaned with normal saline and a bag urine specimen is collected. Results are as follows: $10-100 \times 10^3$ white cells/ml, $10-100 \times 10^3$ red cells/ml, microorganisms seen on Gram stain and a mixed growth of $>100\,000$ coliforms/ml is obtained. Which of the following is/are appropriate?

A Start treatment with co-trimoxazole.
B Repeat bag urine collection.
C Arrange urgent micturating cystogram.
D Collect urine by suprapubic aspiration or clean catch.
E Order aspirin to reduce fever.

10.5. A 2-week-old boy has developed a fever (temperature 38.8°C) and is lethargic. He is noted to be mildly jaundiced. Examination of bag specimen of urine shows on microscopy: red cells $<10 \times 10^3$/ml, white cells $10-100 \times 10^3$/ml, organisms seen and culture of urine showed: $10\,000-100\,000$ coliform organisms/ml, sensitive to all antibiotics tested. Which of the following statements is/are correct?

A Treatment with an appropriate antibiotic should be commenced immediately.
B Blood will show raised conjugated bilirubin.
C Treatment should be withheld until a specimen of urine is obtained by suprapubic bladder aspiration.
D This baby's jaundice is probably related to urinary tract infection.
E Urinary infection at this age is more common in boys than in girls.

10.6. The bacterial colony count in urine from a patient with urinary tract infection may be falsely low in which of the following circumstances?

A As a result of contamination of the specimen with antiseptic.
B After a single dose of trimethoprim with sulphamethoxazole.
C When the urine specific gravity is less than 1.003.
D During prolonged periods of fever.
E When the specimen is an early morning collection.

10.4. D
The microscopic examination of urine in this girl suggests a diagnosis of urinary tract infection,al though the specimen obtained for culture suggests contamination of the specimen. To make a definitive diagnosis a further specimen of urine needs to be examined. In order to ensure there is no contamination it should be obtained by clean catch or suprapubic aspiration. Treatment with co-trimoxazole is not justified without making a definitive diagnosis. A further bag urine sample may also be contaminated, and thus delay treatment. Aspirin is not recommended for treatment of fever in children because it has been implicated in Reye's syndrome.

10.5. B C D E
Microscopic examination of the urine in this child suggests urinary tract infection, although the urine specimen for culture does not completely support the diagnosis. Antibiotic treatment should commence only after another appropriate specimen of urine has been collected, which is best achieved by suprapubic bladder aspiration. In newborn infants there is male sex predilection for urinary tract infection. In this age group jaundice may be the presenting symptom; this is mainly due to raised levels of conjugated bilirubin.

10.6. A B C
Antiseptics used to clean the vulva may inhibit the growth of organisms. Even a single dose of an antibiotic can inhibit growth of organisms. Dilute urine contains fewer organisms per ml than does concentrated urine (found in early morning specimen and fevers).

10.7. Which of the following statements is/are true of urinary tract infection?

A Presence of albumin in the urine establishes the diagnosis.

B The presence of blood in the urine excludes the diagnosis.

C The presence of white blood cells in the urine does not establish the diagnosis.

D Urinary tract infection is more common in circumcised than uncircumcised neonates.

E Single dose antibiotic therapy is not recommended for infants.

10.8. Which of the following statements is/are true of vesicoureteric reflux?

A Young siblings of children with vesicoureteric reflux should be screened.

B Incidence increases with increasing age.

C A normal renal ultrasound appearance in a child of 2 years rules out the possibility of vesicoureteric reflux.

D Renal ultrasonography is the most sensitive imaging modality in the detection of renal scarring (reflux nephropathy).

E Amoxycillin is an appropriate antibiotic for long-term prophylaxis for urinary infection in children with vesicoureteric reflux.

10.9. Which of the following statements is/are true of vesicoureteric reflux and reflux nephropathy?

A Vesicoureteric reflux is best diagnosed by intravenous urography.

B Vesicoureteric reflux is found in more than 50% of all children presenting with urinary tract infection.

C It can cause renal scarring.

D It can result from urinary tract infection.

E Reflux nephropathy only leads to hypertension in the presence of renal failure.

10.10. Which of the following statements is/are true of post-streptococcal glomerulonephritis?

A More than 10% of children develop chronic renal failure.

B Hypertensive encephalopathy is a recognized complication.

C ASO titre is the most useful marker of streptococcal infection.

D Life-long penicillin prophylaxis is recommended.

E Abnormalities of serum complement usually persist for more than 3 months.

10.7. C E

The diagnosis of urinary tract infection can only be established by culture of the urine, although it may be suspected if white blood cells or organisms are seen in urine on microscopy. The presence or absence of albumin and blood are of no significance in urinary tract infection. There is statistical evidence that urinary tract infection is more common in uncircumcised than circumcised neonates. Although single dose therapy has been shown to be efficacious in adults, it is not recommended in infants as complete eradication of infection does not occur.

10.8. A

Familial incidence of vesicoureteric reflux is high. Vesicoureteric reflux is uncommon in later childhood as there is resolution with time. The best way of diagnosing vesicoureteric reflux is by a micturating cystourethrogram. DMSA scan is a more sensitive method of diagnosing renal scarring than renal ultrasonography. Trimethoprim with sulphamethoxazole (Bactrim) but not amoxycillin is the drug of choice for long-term prophylaxis for urinary tract infection in children with vesicoureteric reflux as organisms develop resistance to amoxycillin very rapidly.

10.9. C

Vesicoureteric reflux, a congenital abnormality, is best diagnosed by a micturating cystourethrogram. Its incidence decreases with increasing age. It is found in approximately 30% of all children presenting with urinary tract infection. The incidence of renal scarring increases with the grade of reflux. Reflux nephropathy is the most common cause of hypertension in children with or without renal failure.

10.10. B C

Less than 5% of children with post-streptococcal glomerulonephritis develop chronic renal failure. Complications of acute glomerulonephritis include renal failure, cardiac failure, hypertension and hypertensive encephalopathy. Of the many markers of streptococcal infection, ASO titre is the most useful. Life-long penicillin prophylaxis is not recommended as second attacks of acute glomerulonephritis are rare. Serum complement levels are low only during the acute phase and return to normal within 3 months after the onset of the disease.

10.11. Post-streptococcal acute glomerulonephritis is associated with
A   oliguria.
B   fall in C3 complement levels.
C   rise in serum IgA levels.
D   hypoalbuminaemia.
E   granular and red cell casts in urine.

10.12. A child of 5 years presents with fits and coma. Apart from a sore throat the week before, his previous health has been satisfactory. There is slight facial and peripheral oedema. Examination of the fundi shows bilateral papilloedema. Fine crepitations are heard throughout the lung fields. Blood pressure is 200/120 mmHg. The urine is rusty in colour and stix testing for blood and protein is positive. Serum urea is 25 mmol/l and electrolytes are normal. Haemoglobin is 85 g/l and haematocrit is 0.25. Which of the following statements is/are correct?
A   Fits and coma are due to the elevated blood urea.
B   Anaemia is due to blood loss.
C   Crepitations are due to heart failure.
D   Urgent treatment with anti-hypertensive drugs is indicated.
E   Urgent treatment with steroids is indicated.

10.13. Which of the following statements is/are true of minimal change nephrotic syndrome in childhood?
A   Proteinuria clears within 2 weeks of administration of an adequate course of corticosteroids in at least 75% of cases.
B   Cyclophosphamide can be used to induce prolonged remissions in children with frequent relapses.
C   Red cell casts are found in urine.
D   Oedema is best treated with oral diuretics.
E   Persistent hypertension would be an unexpected finding.

10.11. A B E

There is a fall in C3 fraction of complement because of activation of the alternate pathway. Serum IgA and albumin levels are within normal limits. Urine shows granular and red cell casts. Oliguria occurs in severe cases.

10.12. C D

A history of preceding sore throat (presumably streptococcal), peripheral oedema and papilloedema accompanied by hypertension suggests a diagnosis of post-streptococcal glomerulonephritis complicated by hypertensive encephalopathy. Hypertension rather than raised blood urea is the cause of the fits. Anaemia in acute glomerulonephritis is due to the increase in plasma volume. Patients with acute glomerulonephritis can develop heart failure with or without hypertension. Hypertensive encephalopathy in acute glomerular nephritis can be fatal and requires urgent aggressive treatment to lower the blood pressure. Steroids are of no benefit and could aggravate the hypertension.

10.13. A B E

Proteinuria clears within a period of 2 weeks in more than 75% of cases of nephrotic syndrome. Patients with frequent relapses may respond to treatment with cyclophosphamide. Red blood cell casts in urine are indicative of glomerulonephritis and are not seen in minimal change nephrotic syndrome. Hypertension is unusual. Diuretics are not indicated and may be dangerous because of the decreased plasma volume.

10.14. A 2-year-old boy presents with generalized swelling which has developed over the preceding week. His urine output has diminished considerably during this period. Physical examination reveals generalized pitting oedema. Blood pressure is 100/75 mmHg. Urine contains protein +++, hyaline casts +, no RBC or WBC. He is likely to have

A   raised blood urea.
B   increased susceptibility to pneumococcal infection.
C   low fractional excretion of sodium.
D   selective proteinuria.
E   low levels of serum complement.

10.15. Which of the following features indicate a poor prognosis in children with nephrotic syndrome?

A   Onset before the age of 3 months.
B   Failure of response to treatment with steroids in 4 weeks.
C   More than four relapses in 12 months.
D   Low urinary sodium during relapse.
E   Severity of oedema.

10.16. A 6-year-old boy has transient macroscopic haematuria at the time of an upper respiratory tract infection. He has a past history of haematuria during two similar infections 6 and 10 months earlier. Which of the following statements is/are likely to be true?

A   Renal histology would reveal a focal and/or segmental proliferative glomerulonephritis in about 50% of such cases.
B   Serum IgA levels are likely to be elevated.
C   The serum level of the 3rd component of complement would be normal.
D   He is likely to progress to end-stage renal failure.
E   The antistreptolysin O titre is likely to be raised after an episode of haematuria.

10.17. Which of the following statements concerning chronic renal failure in childhood is/are true?

A   Polyuria may be the presenting symptom.
B   Growth is generally retarded.
C   Anaemia is usually unresponsive to iron, folic acid and Vitamin B_{12}.
D   Normal urinalysis is inconsistent with the diagnosis.
E   Renal transplant is only possible in children more than 5 years of age or more than 20 kg in weight.

10.14. B C D

The history suggests a diagnosis of nephrotic syndrome, in which the blood urea is normal or low, and fractional excretion of sodium is low. There is an increased tendency to pneumococcal infections. The urine shows selective proteinuria (i.e. larger amounts of low molecular weight fractions than of high molecular weight fractions).

10.15. A B

Nephrotic syndrome presenting before the age of 3 months carries a poor prognosis. Patients who do not show a response to corticosteroid up to 4 weeks after commencement of treatment have a poor prognosis as the pathology is usually other than minimal change. Frequent relapses (which are common), low urinary sodium and severity of oedema bear no relationship to the prognosis.

10.16. A C

Recurrent haematuria in a male child associated with respiratory tract infections which are viral supports a diagnosis of IgA nephropathy in which there are focal and/or segmented mesangial proliferative changes in the glomeruli. Serum levels of C3 fraction of complement are not depressed. IgA levels are increased in only 10–15% of cases. The condition does not lead to significant kidney damage in most paediatric patients.

10.17. A B C

Chronic renal failure is characterized by growth failure and anaemia. The latter is due to marrow hypoplasia. Most cases of chronic renal failure in children are due to reflux nephropathy, followed as a close second by congenital malformations. Urine analysis may show no albumin or red blood cells but specific gravity may be low in end-stage renal disease. Rejection of renal transplant is no more frequent in children than in adults. Inability to concentrate urine causes polyuritis.

10.18. Chronic renal failure is seen in association with, or as a sequel to
A Henoch–Schönlein purpura.
B IgA nephropathy.
C vesicoureteric reflux.
D idiopathic thrombocytopenic purpura.
E sickle cell disease.

10.19. Which of the following statements is/are true?
A The percentage of intracellular fluid in the fetus decreases with increasing gestational age.
B The extracellular fluid volume constitutes 20–25% of body weight in the older child.
C The infant of a diabetic mother has an increased percentage of extracellular fluid volume.
D The percentage of extracellular fluid volume tends to decrease with age.
E Total body water represents a smaller percentage of body weight in an obese child than in a normal child.

10.20. Which of the following statements is/are true of oral rehydrating fluids?
A Glucose is essential because it aids in the absorption of electrolytes and water.
B They contain glucose to supply the full caloric needs of the infant.
C The sodium and chloride content of the solution is that of normal saline.
D Sucrose may be substituted for glucose in the solution.
E The infant may continue breastfeeding while receiving oral rehydration fluid.

10.21. Which of the following is/are recognized complications of hypernatraemic dehydration?
A Fits.
B Cardiac arrhythmias.
C Brain damage.
D Hypertension.
E Polyuria.

10.18. A B C E

Henoch–Schönlein purpura, IgA nephropathy and vesicoureteric reflux can all cause chronic renal failure. Idiopathic thrombocytopenic purpura does not affect the kidney. In sickle cell disease end-stage failure occurs as a results of multiple infarcts in the kidney.

10.19. B D E

In the fetus extracellular fluid volume is larger than the intracellular space, but the ratio of extracellular fluid to intracellular fluid falls to the adult level by 9 months of postnatal age. In the older child the volume of extracellular fluid is 20–25% of body weight, compared with 40% at birth. The extracellular fluid volume is contracted in infants of diabetic mothers. Since fat is low in water content, total body water represents a smaller percentage of body weight in an obese than in a normal person.

10.20. A D E

There is active reabsorption of water and electrolytes during the transfer of glucose across the cell membrane. The calories supplied by the glucose in the solution are inadequate. The sodium and chloride content is one-third to one-half normal saline depending on the type of oral rehydrating solution. Sucrose is readily digested, even in infants with severe gastroenteritis, and can be used as a substitute in oral rehydrating solution. Breastfeeding should be allowed in breast-fed infants and water should be offered *ad lib* to other infants.

10.21. A C

Hypernatraemic dehydration causes fits during rehydration therapy as a result of brain swelling. Cerebral palsy may result from sagittal sinus thrombosis. Cardiac arrhythmias, hypertension and polyuria are not seen.

10.22. In hypernatraemic dehydration complicating gastroenteritis
A   there is no potassium loss.
B   there is no sodium loss.
C   intracellular water is preserved.
D   isotonic fluids are required for intravenous rehydration.
E   there is a risk of seizures.

10.23. Potassium
A   is the main intracellular cation of the body.
B   depletion commonly causes diarrhoea.
C   is mainly reabsorbed in the proximal tubule.
D   is mainly excreted in stool.
E   serum levels are sensitive to small changes in total body potassium.

10.24. Acute deficiency of potassium may produce
A   tall peaked T waves in the ECG.
B   muscle weakness.
C   ileus.
D   nystagmus.
E   abdominal distension.

10.25. Hypokalaemia is likely to occur in
A   diarrhoea.
B   renal tubular acidosis.
C   infants of diabetic mothers.
D   infantile pyloric stenosis.
E   neonatal asphyxia.

10.26. Metabolic acidosis is seen in children under which of the following circumstances?
A   Chronic asthma.
B   Hypertrophic pyloric stenosis.
C   Diabetes mellitus.
D   Gastroenteritis.
E   Peripheral circulatory failure.

10.22. D E
In hypernatraemic dehydration there is loss of electrolytes and water but the water loss is greater. As a result of the hyernatraemia, intracellular water moves from the cells to the extracellular compartment. It is important to administer isotonic fluids in order to prevent rapid movement of the water back into the cells, which may result in cerebral oedema and seizures.

10.23. A C
Intracellular concentrations of potassium approximate 150 mmol/l. Almost all of the filtered potassium is reabsorbed in the proximal renal tubule. Although diarrhoea may cause potassium depletion, potassium depletion causes ileus. Very small amounts of potassium are normally excreted in the stool as most of it is reabsorbed in the gut. As the vast majority of total body potassium is in the intracellular fluid, serum levels are not sensitive to small changes in total body potassium.

10.24. B C E
Hypokalaemia produces functional alterations in muscle which results in lower T wave in ECG, muscle paralysis and ileus which would cause abdominal distension. There is no nystagmus.

10.25. A B D
As gastrointestinal fluids contain large quantitites of potassium, their loss in diarrhoea and infantile pyloric stenosis results in hypokalaemia. In pyloric stenosis loss of hydrogen ion as a result of vomiting leads to increased loss of potassium in the urine (hydrogen ion is exchanged for potassium ion in the distal renal tubule) which further aggravates the problem. In renal tubular acidosis the hypokalaemia is due to loss of potassium in the urine. In neonatal asphyxia potassium leaks out of the cells resulting in hyperkalaemia. There is no disturbance of serum potassium in infants of diabetic mothers.

10.26. C D E
Chronic asthma results in respiratory acidosis as a result of carbon dioxide retention. In hypertrophic pyloric stenosis loss of chloride and hydrogen ions leads to metabolic alkalosis. In diabetes mellitus there is increase in ketone bodies resulting in metabolic acidosis. In gastroenteritis there is loss of bicarbonate in the stools resulting in metabolic acidosis. In peripheral circulatory failure there is accumulation of lactic acid due to anaerobic metabolism in tissues.

190

10.27. Alkalosis may be a problem in
A   infantile gastroenteritis.
B   neonatal duodenal obstruction.
C   hyaline membrane disease.
D   pyloric stenosis.
E   starvation.

10.28. The following is a report of blood gas analysis in a newborn infant (receiving oxygen therapy) with respiratory difficulty: pH 7.35, Pco_2 30 mmHg, Po_2 60 mmHg. The infant
A   has respiratory alkalosis.
B   has compensated metabolic acidosis.
C   requires treatment with sodium bicarbonate.
D   needs more oxygen.
E   requires no change in management.

10.29. A 1-year-old infant has diarrhoea and vomiting for 3 days. The infant's temperature is 39°C and he is very irritable. Very little urine being passed but there are no other signs of dehydration. Mother says that she has been feeding full-strength skimmed milk since the commencement of the illness. Which of the following statements is/are correct?
A   Hypernatraemia is likely to be found.
B   The infant should be given 300 ml of 5% dextrose rapidly.
C   The infant is at risk of developing cerebral palsy.
D   Dehydration should be corrected over 48 h.
E   The infant is not dehydrated.

10.30. In inappropriate ADH secretion
A   urinary osmolality is higher than serum osmolality.
B   urinary output is decreased.
C   the patient is hypovolaemic.
D   ADH secretion is decreased.
E   total body sodium is decreased.

10.27. B D
Infantile gastroenteritis results in metabolic acidosis due to loss of bicarbonate. Neonatal duodenal obstruction and pyloric stenosis result in alkalosis because of loss of gastric acid juice. Hyaline membrane disease results in a mixed respiratory (raised carbon dioxide tension) and metabolic (anaerobic metabolism) acidosis. Starvation results in ketoacidosis.

10.28. B E
A pH of 7.35 with a low P_{CO_2} (30 mmHg) indicates metabolic acidosis. As the acid–base disturbance is minimal and the P_{O_2} is normal for the age, no change in management is indicated.

10.29. A C D
The presence of diarrhoea, vomiting and scanty urine indicates that the patient is dehydrated. Full-strength skimmed milk is high in electrolytes which will result in hypernatraemia. In such infants the dehydration should be corrected slowly by administration of fluids containing normal or half-normal saline as rapid fluid administration will result in cerebral oedema.

10.30. A B E
In inappropriate ADH secretion the patient passes small quantities of concentrated urine due to increased ADH secretion which causes retention of fluid leading to hyponatraemia. The plasma concentration of atrial natriuretic peptide is increased which is the major factor in the natriuresis of inappropriate ADH (despite the hyponatremia) which results in negative sodium balance.

11 Endocrinology and gonads

11.1. Growth hormone secretion in normal individuals is stimulated by which of the following?
A Exercise.
B Hydrocortisone.
C Arginine infusion.
D Insulin-induced hypoglycaemia.
E Sleep.

11.2. Output of growth hormone can be reduced by
A psychosocial deprivation.
B hypoglycaemia.
C exercise.
D sleep.
E malnutrition.

11.3. Congenital hypothyroidism
A is less common than phenylketonuria.
B is reliably detected by biochemical investigation in the first week of life.
C is reliably detected by clinical examination in the first week of life.
D is commonly associated with other endocrine deficiencies.
E can cause delay in bone maturation.

11.4. Which of the following is/are likely to be associated with juvenile hypothyroidism presenting at the age of 8 years?
A Ectopic thyroid.
B Athyreosis.
C Obesity.
D Constipation.
E Malformed epiphyses.

11.1. A C D E
Growth hormone secretion is stimulated by sleep, exercise, arginine infusion and hypoglycaemia. Hydrocortisone does not stimulate growth hormone secretion.

11.2. A E
Growth hormone production is reduced in psychosocial deprivation and malnutrition but this is not a constant feature in these conditions. Growth hormone production is often increased during hypoglycaemia, exercise and sleep.

11.3. B E
The incidence of congenital hypothyroidism is 1 in 4000, while that of phenylketonuria is 1 in 14000. Careful evaluation of TSH and T4 will establish the diagnosis. There are few reliable physical signs in the first week of life. Congenital hypothyroidism is usually an isolated defect. Bone age is delayed.

11.4. D E
Constipation and malformed epiphyses are classical physical findings in juvenile hypothyroidism. The thyroid gland is always present and is usually not ectopic. Obesity is uncommon.

11.5. Guide(s) to the diagnosis of hypothyroidism in the newborn is/are
A   hypothermia.
B   conjugated hyperbilirubinaemia.
C   radiographic signs of delay in osseous development.
D   low birth weight for period of gestation.
E   hyperglycaemia.

11.6. A 14-year-old girl has a smooth, non-tender goitre without any other symptoms. Investigations show T4 87 ng/l (normal 85–160), TSH 11 ng/l (normal 2–3.5) and antimicrosomal antibody titre 1/12 500 (normal less than 1/100). Which of the following statements is/are correct?
A   She has compensated hypothyroidism.
B   This presentation of thyroid disease is rare in teenage children.
C   Spontaneous remission of this condition has been observed.
D   Other endocrine abnormalities may also be found.
E   The most likely diagnosis is Graves' disease.

11.7. Enlargement of the thyroid gland may be produced by
A   a deficient intake of iodine.
B   craniopharyngioma.
C   growth hormone.
D   pregnancy.
E   autoimmune disease.

11.8. Which of the following statements is/are true?
A   Propylthiouracil crosses the placenta.
B   Thyroid-stimulating antibodies (TSI) cross the placenta.
C   In untreated hypothyroid children, the legs are disproportionately shorter than the head and trunk.
D   Neonatal hypothyroidism may present as persistent jaundice.
E   Early diagnosis and treatment of congenital hypothyroidism prevents delay in development in most cases.

11.5. A C
Hypothyroidism may present with hypothermia at any age. The other symptom in the neonatal period is prolonged hyperbilirubinaemia, but the bilirubin is not conjugated. X-rays of the knee and ankle show delayed bone age. Newborn infants are normal or large for gestation. Infants with hypothyroidism may present with hypoglycaemia but not hyperglycaemia.

11.6. A C D
A raised TSH level in the presence of low normal T4 levels supports a diagnosis of compensated hypothyroidism. This is most commonly due to Hashimoto thyroiditis in teenage girls. The diagnosis is confirmed by the presence of thyroid antibodies. The goitre has been observed to resolve spontaneously. Clinical manifestations of Hashimoto disease include goitre (which may be euthyroid, hypothyroid or thyrotoxic) and may be associated with other autoimmune diseases such as diabetes mellitus, adrenal insufficiency, hypoparathyroidism and, less commonly, pernicious anaemia and thrombocytopenia.

11.7. A D E
Lack of iodine causes hypertrophy of the acinar tissue and enlargement of the thyroid gland. Craniopharyngioma may cause a decrease in TSH production and therefore atrophy of the thyroid gland. Growth hormone does not effect thyroid size. Lymphocytic thyroiditis, which is an autoimmune disease, is the most common cause of goitre in childhood. There is an increase in size of the thyroid gland during pregnancy.

11.8. A B C D E
Propylthiouracil crosses the placenta and may cause congenital hypothyroidism. Thyroid-stimulating immune globulins cross the placenta and may cause hyperthyroidism in newborn infants (even though the mother may have no signs of hyperthyroidism). Long bones do not grow in untreated hypothyroid children. In neonatal hypothyroidism the jaundice is prolonged. Early treatment of congenital hypothyroidism prevents mental retardation.

11.9. Which of the following statements is/are true of the thyroid-stimulating hormone (TSH) level in capillary blood of newborn infants?
A   Levels are elevated in congenital hypothyroidism.
B   It will detect pituitary hypothyroidism.
C   It measures TSH produced by the infant.
D   It is suitable for mass screening.
E   It is increased in the presence of maternal Hashimoto thyroiditis.

11.10. Recognized complications of long-term therapy with prednisolone in childhood include
A   growth retardation.
B   postural hypotension.
C   exacerbation of fungal infection.
D   proximal myopathy.
E   peripheral neuropathy.

11.11. Congenital adrenal hyperplasia (21-hydroxylase deficiency)
A   is associated with high plasma 17-hydroxyprogesterone levels.
B   is a common cause of ambiguous genitalia in newborn girls.
C   may be associated with salt wasting.
D   is associated with high plasma cortisol levels.
E   may be complicated by infertility.

11.12. Which of the following statements is/are true?
A   Congenital adrenal hyperplasia may present as masculinization of a female newborn.
B   In congenital adrenal hyperplasia there is often a salt-losing state.
C   In testicular feminization syndrome the gonads secrete testosterone, but there is a failure of end organ response.
D   Growth hormone deficiency results in disproportionate shortening of the lower limbs.
E   In diabetes insipidus, urine output and fluid intake are influenced by the dietary solute load.

11.9. A C D
In congenital hypothyroidism capillary blood of the newborn shows elevated levels of TSH. In pituitary hypothyroidism both TSH and FT_4/T_3 are low. TSH does not cross the placenta. It is suitable for mass screening of primary hypothyroidism. Maternal Hashimoto's thyroiditis does not affect the infant's TSH.

11.10. A C D
Corticosteroids cause growth retardation, hypertension, predisposition to infection and myopathy in children.

11.11. A B C E
Plasma 17-hydroxy progesterone levels are high in congenital adrenal hyperplasia. The plasma cortisol levels are normal or low. CAH should be considered in the differential diagnosis of ambiguous genitalia in the newborn and may present with low serum sodium (due to salt loss in the urine) and hyperkalaemia. Infertility is a complication of poor control during puberty.

11.12. A B C E
In newborn female infants the masculinization is due to blockage of the pathway to the formation of hydrocortisone which results in the increased formation of androgens. The salt-losing state is not always present. In testicular feminization syndrome the patient is phenotypically female, although the gonads are testes and there is no uterus. The testes produce testosterone which suggests that there is failure of end organ response. Growth hormone deficiency does not cause abnormal body proportions. In diabetes insipidus, water turnover is directly proportional to the obligatory renal solute presented in the diet.

11.13. A female infant is born with virilization of the external genitalia. Plasma 17-hydroxyprogesterone and ACTH levels are elevated. Which of the following statements is/are true?

A Congenital adrenal hyperplasia is the most likely diagnosis.
B The baby would have normal internal genitalia.
C The mother has been treated with progestogens.
D A salt-losing tendency may be present in this infant.
E The bone age may be normal.

11.14. Which of the following is/are true of diabetes mellitus with onset in the first decade?

A It usually occurs in obese children.
B There is an increase in insulin requirements at puberty.
C Less insulin is required when appetite is reduced due to acute infections.
D It should not be treated with oral hypoglycaemic agents.
E Competitive games should be avoided.

11.15. Which of the following statements is/are true about diabetes mellitus in childhood?

A Congenital rubella is a recognized cause.
B It is a frequent cause of adult blindness.
C It may present with acute abdominal pain.
D The concordance rate among monozygotic twins is about 50%.
E There is good correlation between blood glucose control and HbA_{1C} levels.

11.16. In the education of a diabetic which of the following statements is/are appropriate?

A Routine blood glucose should be measured before every injection of short-acting insulin.
B For prevention of nocturnal hypoglycaemia blood glucose should be tested intermittently at 2–3 a.m.
C Adjustments for anticipated change in physical activity can be made by altering the dietary schedule or the insulin dose.
D Headaches upon awakening may be due to nocturnal hypoglycaemia.
E Rapid-acting insulin doses should be given on a sliding scale according to blood glucose results.

11.13. A B D E
The clinical presentation and laboratory findings support the diagnosis of adrenal hyperplasia, which may have a salt-losing tendency. Bone age is normal in spite of excess intrauterine androgen exposure. However, bone age is increased postnatally in untreated cases. Maternal progestogens can cause masculinization, but in these cases adrenal function is normal at birth.

11.14. B D
Juvenile diabetes has no relationship with obesity. Insulin requirements increase at puberty. Acute infections increase the requirements of insulin. Juvenile diabetes should not be treated with oral hypoglycaemic agents as there is an absolute lack of insulin production by the pancreas. No restrictions should be placed on activity when the condition is well-controlled.

11.15. A B C D E
Congenital rubella is a recognized cause of diabetes mellitus. Juvenile diabetes mellitus leads to diabetic retinopathy and blindness in adults. Diabetic keto-acidosis is a recognized cause of acute abdominal pain. Though heredity has been implicated in type 1 diabetes mellitus, environmental factors are important: even in monozygotic twins the concordance rate is about 50%. The blood and urine sugar levels do not correlate well. HbA_{1C} is a good indicator of control of diabetes mellitus over the preceding 4–10 weeks.

11.16. A B C D E
The young diabetic should be taught to measure blood glucose. He should measure it before injecting short-acting insulin and be able to adjust the dosage depending on blood glucose levels. He should also be advised on how to adjust the insulin dosage with changes in physical activity and dietary intake. He should be made aware that nocturnal hypoglycaemia, which may be prevented by knowledge of blood glucose levels at 2 and 3 a.m., can present as headache on awakening.

11.17. A 4-year-old boy presents with drowsiness, hyperpnoea and vomiting. He has been unwell for several days. Acetone can be smelt on his breath and the urine contains sugar in large quantities. Other clinical signs and symptoms associated with this disorder include
A   antecedent increase in thirst.
B   antecedent weight loss.
C   moderate to severe dehydration.
D   constipation.
E   Kussmaul breathing (deep sighing respiraticn).

11.18. A young boy, known to be a diabetic taking insulin, is found unconscious at 11.00 a.m. His mother reports that he went off to school quite well about 8.00 a.m. that morning. You would expect to find
A   hyperventilation.
B   blood glucose below 3.0 mmol/l.
C   ketone bodies in the urine.
D   a good response to injected glucagon.
E   sweating.

11.19. In which of the following may glucose appear in the urine?
A   Fanconi syndrome.
B   Congenital adrenal hyperplasia.
C   Cerebral haemorrhage.
D   Galactosaemia.
E   Salicylate intoxication.

11.20. Low blood glucose may be found in
A   low birth weight for gestational age infants.
B   Cushing syndrome.
C   glycogen storage disease.
D   galactosaemia.
E   alcohol ingestion.

11.17. A B C D E
The stem suggests a diagnosis of juvenile diabetes mellitus. All the distractors are symptoms which may be found in this condition.

11.18. B D E
The history supports a diagnosis of insulin-induced hypoglycaemia. Hyperventilation, which is due to acidosis, is a feature of diabetic ketosis. Hypoglycaemic patients do not hyperventilate, their blood glucose is low and sweating is a common symptom. Ketone bodies are not usually present in the urine. As an insulin antagonist, glucagon will increase the blood glucose.

11.19. A C E
In Fanconi syndrome there is glycosuria and aminoaciduria. Cerebral haemorrhage and salicylate intoxication cause hyperglycaemia leading to glycosuria. There is no glycosuria in congenital adrenal hyperplasia. In galactosaemia urine contains reducing substances (galactose) but no glucose.

11.20. A C D E
The low blood sugar in infants with a low birth weight for gestational age is due to low glycogen and gluconeogenic reserves; in galactosaemia it is due to liver failure as a result of damage to the liver and in glycogen storage disease due to the absence of enzymes which break down glycogen. In Cushing syndrome there is hyperglycaemia. Alcohol ingestion causes suppression of hepatic gluconeogenesis and reduction of glucose output by the liver.

11.21. Which of the following statements is/are true of inappropriate ADH?
A   The serum sodium concentration is low.
B   Urinary output is diminished.
C   Fluid intake should be restricted.
D   Patients with fits require hypertonic saline.
E   Urinary sodium concentration is low.

11.22. Which of the following statements is/are true?
A   The prepuce cannot be gently retracted in more than 20% of boys by the age of 1 year.
B   Phimosis following balanitis is an indication for circumcision.
C   Circumcision before the child is out of nappies increases the risk of meatal ulcer.
D   If the prepuce cannot be retracted by the age of 5 years, the child needs circumcision.
E   There is no medical indication for circumcision in the newborn infant.

11.23. Which of the following statements is/are true of penile hypospadias?
A   The chordee is often the major functional disability.
B   The urethral meatus is often very narrow.
C   Urethral sphincter is often deficient.
D   Impotence is present in more than 20% of cases.
E   Neonatal circumcision is absolutely contraindicated.

11.24. Torsion of a testis
A   is caused by an anatomic abnormality.
B   is rare before puberty.
C   may cause sterility if it is bilateral.
D   requires exploration of the contralateral testis
E   is rarely precipitated by exertion or trauma.

11.21. A B C D
Inappropriate ADH secretion occurs in a number of unrelated conditions, including CNS infections and trauma, respiratory problems, drug treatment (vincristine) and malignant tumours (pancreas, Ewing sarcoma). The serum sodium (and osmolality) is low whereas excretion of sodium in urine is continued. Urine output is diminished. Treatment consists of restriction of fluids and management of the primary condition. Hypertonic saline should be reserved for patients with neurological symptoms.

11.22. A C E
At birth less than 5% of normal boys have a fully retractable prepuce. By the age of 3 years the prepuce can be retracted in 90% of boys. Complications such as haemorrhage and infection are more likely to occur in the first week of life. Ammoniacal dermatitis is the commonest cause of meatal ulcer. Unless definite phimosis is present circumcision is not indicated at any age, even though there is evidence that urinary tract infection occurs significantly more commonly in uncircumcised infants.

11.23. A B E
In penile hypospadias the chordee prevents the child from passing urine in the standing position as it would wet his legs. Although the urethra may be normal the meatus is often stenotic. Neonatal circumcision is contraindicated as the foreskin is needed for repair later. There is no abnormality of the sphincters. Although sexual intercourse may be difficult, there is no impotence.

11.24. A C D
Torsion of the testis is caused by abnormal fixation of the gonad as the tunica vaginalis covers not only the testis but the epididymis and the spermatic cord as well. The majority of torsions occur before the age of 6 years and result in destruction of the gonad unless immediate treatment is initiated. Since the anatomical abnormality is usually bilateral, the contralateral testis should be explored and fixed. There is no evidence that trauma plays any role in the aetiology of torsion of the testis.

11.25. Which of the following statements is/are true of undescended testes?
A   The average age at full descent is 1 year.
B   Retractile testes should be surgically fixed in the scrotum.
C   The testes are undescended at birth in more than 50% of male infants of less than 1500 g.
D   Ectopic testes should be excised.
E   An undescended testis should be brought down by operation by the age of 2 years.

11.26. Which of the following is/are more likely to occur in a patient with undescended testes?
A   Trauma to the testes.
B   Infertility.
C   Torsion of the testes.
D   Malignancy of the testes.
E   Testicular dysplasia.

11.27. Which of the following statements is/are correct?
A   A retractile testis may be found in the inguinal canal.
B   The cremasteric reflex is most active between the ages of 6 months and 4 years.
C   In unilateral cryptorchidism the undescended testis is usually larger than the descended one.
D   More than 50% of undescended testis diagnosed at birth descend by the age of 1 year.
E   Malignancy is unlikely to occur in an undescended testis before the age of 5 years.

11.28. Adherent labia minora
A   usually indicate an underlying vaginal atresia.
B   can cause acute urinary retention.
C   can be treated by the application of an oestrogen cream.
D   require reconstructive surgery for the girl to conceive normally.
E   are rarely associated with urogenital problems.

11.25. C E

The testis begins to descend at 28 weeks' gestation and is in the scrotum by 34 weeks' gestation (2 kg) in the majority of cases. Retractile testes retract into the inguinal canal in response to an exaggerated cremasteric reflex. They can be brought down by careful manipulation when the child is relaxed in a warm room. Ectopic testes are morphologically normal and therefore should not be excised. Most undescended testes that are likely to descend will do so by the end of the first year. Dysplastic changes are detectable in the testis by the end of the first year and continue to increase thereafter.

11.26. A B C D E

The undescended testis is dysplastic and atrophic which results in infertility. The risk of malignancy is 20–40% more than in the normal testis. As the testis may be in the inguinal region there is an increased risk of trauma and torsion.

11.27. A B D E

The cremasteric reflex is weak or absent at birth and is most active between the ages of 6 months to 4 years. It is not abnormal for the testis to retract into the inguinal canal. Such testes adopt a permanent scrotal position at puberty. The undescended testis is usually atrophic and smaller than the descended one. The incidence of undescended testes in full-term infants at birth is 3–4% compared with 1% at 1 year. Although the incidence of malignancy in the adult population is increased by 40%, testicular malignancy in children under the age of 5 years is extremely rare.

11.28. C E

Adherent labia minora are common and do not have any underlying gynaecological pathology. They cause no symptoms and respond to treatment with topical oestrogens.

11.29. Primary spasmodic dysmenorrhoea is associated with
A   maternal history of the same disorder.
B   anovulation.
C   increased levels of prostaglandins in menstrual blood.
D   irregular menstrual cycle.
E   endometrial hyperplasia.

11.30. Which of the following statements is/are correct regarding abnormal or ambiguous genitalia in a newborn?
A   Hypoglycaemia in a neonate with micropenis should raise suspicion of hypopituitarism.
B   Functioning ovaries are required for normal fetal development of the female genital tract.
C   Gender assignment of a neonate with ambiguous genitalia should be considered an emergency.
D   The presence of testes does not dictate male gender assignment.
E   Hypospadias without palpable testes in a newborn should be investigated.

11.31. Which of the following statements is/are true of sexual development in the fetus?
A   Female genital development does not require gonads.
B   The *sry* gene is necessary for the development of the testis.
C   Testosterone is necessary for the development of vas deferens, epididymis and seminal vesicles.
D   In the male, Müllarian ducts differentiate into vas deferens, epididymis and seminal vesicles.
E   In the female, Müllarian ducts differentiate into Fallopian tubes, uterus and upper part of vagina.

11.29. A C
Primary dysmenorrhoea is caused by myometrial contraction due to high levels of prostaglandin F_2 and E_2 produced by the endometrium. The condition is familial. Ovulation, menstrual cycle and the endometrium (histology) are normal.

11.30. A C D E
Neonatal hypoglycaemia with micropenis has been observed in aplasia of the pituitary gland with no other abnormalities. In the female, development of uterus, ovary and vagina does not require hormones. Gender assignment is largely based on the possibilities for correction of the ambiguous genitalia and not on the gonadal or chromosomal constitution. Hypospadias without palpable testis can be due to anomalies in sexual differentiation in both sexes. Gender assignment at birth is a social emergency.

11.31. A B C E
In the female, genital development is passive. Atrophy of the Wolffian ducts and development of internal female genital organs (from the Müllarian ducts) occurs independent of hormonal stimulation or genetic influences. In the male, the *sry* gene, which is located on chromosome Yp, leads to differentiation of the testis. The testis produces anti-Müllarian hormone (which causes involution of the Müllarian ducts) and testosterone under the influence of which internal male genital organs develop from the Wolffian ducts.

12 Neurology and neurosurgery

12.1. Which of the following statements is/are true of cerebral palsy?

A   There has been a decrease in incidence in the last decade.
B   There is progressive neurological deterioration.
C   There is spontaneous improvement in motor function in some cases.
D   Mental retardation is present in more than 95% of cases.
E   Affected infants may have abnormal tonic neck patterns in the neonatal period.

12.2. A baby boy was born at 32 weeks' gestation. He smiled at 6 weeks and could pick up a small object with finger and thumb at 10 months. He is not yet walking at the age of 26 months. His speech is normal. Likely diagnoses is/are

A   mental subnormality.
B   cerebral palsy.
C   muscular dystrophy.
D   spina bifida occulta.
E   phenylketonuria.

12.3. A 3-year-old boy is found to be functioning at an 18-month level across all areas of development. History (including family history) and physical examination are unremarkable. Which of the following statements is/are true?

A   There is a greater than 75% chance that thorough investigation will reveal a cause.
B   The cerebral CT scan will be abnormal in more than 20% of such children.
C   The serum creatine kinase should be measured.
D   A chromosome study may show X-linked intellectual handicap to be the cause.
E   This child would not qualify for a handicapped child allowance until he reaches school age.

12.4. In complex partial seizures (psychomotor seizures, temporal lobe epilepsy) which of the following may occur as seizure manifestations?

A   Repeated swallowing.
B   Dream-like states.
C   Central abdominal pain.
D   Vertigo.
E   Oculogyric crises.

12.1. C E

The incidence of cerebral palsy has not decreased (it may even have increased because more premature infants with neurological problems are being saved) over the last decade. It is a static lesion, although it may appear to be progressive because the symptoms may not manifest until later. Spontaneous improvement in motor function has been observed, particularly in premature infants. Intelligence may be normal but may be difficult to assess because of disturbed motor function. Obligatory tonic neck patterns may be the only sign in the neonatal period.

12.2. B C

In all areas other than gross motor ability the child is developing normally. He cannot have mental subnormality or phenylketonuria (which causes mental deficiency). Spina bifida occulta does not cause motor problems. Cerebral palsy and muscular dystrophy are possible diagnoses.

12.3. C D

If a diagnosis of mental deficiency cannot be established on history and physical examination the chances of it being diagnosed following investigations are small. The majority of patients with mental deficiency have a morphologically normal brain. Twenty-five percent of children with Duchenne muscular dystrophy (diagnosed by measuring serum creatine kinase) have mental deficiency. In morphologically normal boys X-linked mental retardation is the most common recognizable cause of mental deficiency. The child is eligible for a handicapped child allowance at the age of diagnosis (if applicable).

12.4. A B C D

Complex partial seizures are due to epileptic discharges in the temporal lobes. Symptoms include confusion at the time of the attack without complete loss of consciousness, déjà vu dreamy states, visual and auditory hallucinations, mood disturbances (fear, anxiety, laughing, anger and aggression) and semi-purposeful motor activities (motor automatisms, particularly repeated chewing and swallowing). Central abdominal pain (abdominal epilepsy) and vertigo are other manifestations. Oculogyric crisis do not occur.

12.5. Infantile spasms
A   characteristically occur in the first year of life.
B   are sometimes associated with a characteristic pattern on EEG.
C   may occur in children with tuberous sclerosis.
D   sometimes occur in previously normal children.
E   are a benign seizure disorder.

12.6. Which of the following statements is/are true of simple febrile convulsions?
A   The IQ of children with recurrent febrile convulsions is lower than that of their unaffected siblings.
B   There is an increased risk of recurrence if the first fit occurs before the age of 1 year.
C   An EEG is not indicated in the assessment for treatment of febrile convulsions.
D   The risk of developing epilepsy later is 10 times that of the general population.
E   Phenobarbitone should be administered regularly to all infants with febrile convulsions until the age of 3 years.

12.7. The frequency of recurrence of benign febrile convulsions in childhood can be reduced by
A   prophylactic administration of adequate doses of phenytoin sodium.
B   prophylactic administration of adequate doses of phenobarbital.
C   prophylactic administration of adequate doses of sodium valproate.
D   administration of carbamazepine during febrile illnesses.
E   administration of diazepam rectally regularly during febrile illnesses.

12.8. Some anticonvulsants may produce unwanted side effects when dosage and serum levels are within the recommended range. Which of the following examples illustrate this phenomenon?
A   Phenytoin and diplopia.
B   Oral diazepam and neonatal jaundice.
C   Sodium valproate and liver toxicity.
D   Carbamazepine and Stevens–Johnson syndrome.
E   Phenobarbitone and hyperactivity.

12.5. A B C D
The usual age of onset of infantile spasms is 3–6 months, but they may begin as early as the neonatal period or as late as 2 years. They most commonly occur in association with neonatal asphyxia, birth trauma or previous meningitis. They are also seen in patients with tuberous sclerosis and may sometimes occur in previously normal children. Whooping cough vaccine has also been implicated, but the incidence is less than 1:150 000. Although they may remit spontaneously, other seizure types develop later in life in about 50% of patients and mental retardation has been reported in 80–90% of cases on long-term follow-up. The EEG changes when present are diagnostic (hypsarrhythmia).

12.6. B C
Febrile convulsions do not affect the IQ of children. The EEG is of little or no value in the assessment. The risk of developing epilepsy later is 2–3 times greater than that of the general population. Phenobarbitone is administered regularly to infants who have three or more febrile convulsions but may have to be replaced with sodium valproate if side effects (hyperactivity) occur. The risk is increased if the first fit occurs before the age of 1 year.

12.7. B C E
Controlled trials have shown that prophylactic administration of phenobarbital, sodium valproate and administration of diazepam rectally during febrile illnesses reduces the frequency of occurrence of febrile convulsions. Phenytoin sodium and carbamazepine do not alter the frequency of febrile convulsions.

12.8. C D E
Central nervous system manifestations are most common with phenytoin (Dilantin) overdosage and include diplopia, nystagmus, ataxia, slurred speech and mental confusion. They are due to the direct toxic effect of the drug. Gingival hypertrophy occurs even when the drug is given in therapeutic dosages. Other toxic effects are skin rashes and bone marrow depression which are due to hypersensitivity. Initially, phenobarbitone causes drowsiness; this resolves spontaneously but hyperactivity may be troublesome even with therapeutic dosages. Sodium valproate causes liver toxicity, particularly in the first 2–12 weeks after commencement of therapy. It is thought to be an idiosyncratic response. Carbamazepine therapy results in Stevens–Johnson syndrome in 3% of patients as a result of hypersensitivity. The sodium benzoate included in parenteral diazepam interferes with the binding of bilirubin to albumin; this is not a problem when diazepam is given orally.

12.9. Which of the following statements is/are true of benign febrile convulsions?
A   The diagnosis is not acceptable if the infant is less than 6 months of age.
B   The temperature is usually below 38°C.
C   There is increased incidence in patients with cerebral palsy.
D   The incidence is increased in siblings.
E   There are no focal signs following the seizure.

12.10. Childhood absence (petit mal) epilepsy
A   has a characteristic aura preceding an attack.
B   commonly responds to treatment with ethosuximide.
C   has characteristic 3/s spike and wave discharge patterns on EEG.
D   characteristically commences between 4 and 10 years.
E   is caused by the pertussis component in triple antigen (DPT).

12.11. Which of the following statements is/are true of childhood absence epilepsy (petit mal)?
A   The presenting symptom may be poor school performance.
B   It results in loss of motor activity.
C   Postural tone is not usually affected.
D   The presence of grand mal seizures in the patient excludes such a diagnosis.
E   The drug of choice for treatment is phenytoin sodium.

12.12. An 18-month-old child on three occasions, each after minor trauma, has had episodes in which he has stiffened, become pale, given a cry, fallen on the ground, arched his back, rolled his eyes up and jerked, then has become limp, woken up and, although a little groggy for a few minutes, he then fully recovered. Which of the following is/are correct of this patient?
A   He does not have epilepsy.
B   These attacks require investigations with CT scan, EEG and lumbar puncture.
C   This is a breath holding attack which the child is doing deliberately and ought to be punished.
D   These attacks are breath holding attacks and, to avoid brain damage, mouth-to-mouth resuscitation should be applied in any further attacks.
E   These attacks are syncopal (vasovagal, pale, breath holding) and though alarming they cause no damage.

12.9. A D E

By definition, febrile convulsions occur in normal children over the age of 6 months and under the age of 5 years. The convulsions may occur at any temperature but usually at above 38.5C. There are no changes in the cerebrospinal fluid. There is increased familial incidence and there are no focal signs following the seizure.

12.10. B C D

The drug of choice for treatment of petit mal epilepsy is ethosuximide. It also responds to treatment with valproic acid and tridione. It commences between 4 and 10 years and is characterized by staring and arrest of activity. The EEG shows the characteristic 3/s spike and wave pattern. There is rarely an aura preceding an attack and it has no relationship to pertussis vaccine.

12.11. A B C

Repeated attacks of petit mal epilepsy will result in inattention and poor school performance. During an attack there is sudden brief arrest of motor activity associated with a blank stare without loss of motor tone. Some children with petit mal epilepsy also have concomitant grand mal seizures. The drug of choice for treatment is ethosuximide.

12.12. A E

The history suggests a child with vasovagal attacks with seizures which are not epileptic. They do not require investigation or treatment. They are not deliberate and punishment will not resolve the problem.

12.13. Which of the following is/are true of bacterial meningitis in an 11-month-old infant?
A   The organism can usually be recovered from blood.
B   Neck stiffness may not be present.
C   It often presents with lethargy and refusal to feed.
D   Inappropriate antidiuretic hormone secretion is a recognized feature.
E   Subdural effusions are a recognized complication.

12.14. A 3-year-old boy presents with high fever, irritability and progressive loss of consciousness. Examination shows left VIth nerve palsy, bilateral papilloedema and right hemiparesis. Which of the following statements is/are true?
A   Immediate lumbar puncture is required.
B   The EEG would be abnormal.
C   Blood culture is indicated.
D   CAT scan is indicated.
E   Head ultrasound will establish the diagnosis.

12.15. Recognized causes of deafness include
A   meningitis.
B   chloroquine.
C   aminoglycosides.
D   neonatal hyperbilirubinaemia.
E   sulphadiazine.

12.16. Convergent squint
A   is less common than divergent squint in children.
B   is often associated with hypermetropia.
C   may be completely reversed by the use of spectacles.
D   often resolves spontaneously at the age of about 5 years.
E   is clinically significant principally because of its cosmetic effects.

12.13. A B C D E
Physical signs of meningitis, viz. neck stiffness, Kernig's sign and bulging fontanelle, may not be present in infants. The younger the infant the more likely it is to present with lethargy and refusal to feed. In more than 50% of cases of meningitis the organism can be cultured from blood. Subdural effusions occur during the course of treatment and may require drainage in some cases. Inappropriate antidiuretic hormone secretion often occurs and is manifested by hyponatraemia. It is treated by restriction of fluids.

12.14. B C D
The history and physical examination suggest a diagnosis of a space-occupying lesion with raised intracranial pressure in the left hemisphere, possibly associated with infection. Lumbar puncture is dangerous as it may cause herniation of the medulla. The EEG would be abnormal and a CAT scan would accurately demonstrate the position and the nature of the lesion. Head ultrasound, though helpful, is not possible (fonantelle being closed) and therefore will not establish the diagnosis.

12.15. A C D
Neonatal hyperbilirubinaemia and aminoglycosides cause sensorineural hearing loss. Complications of meningitis include cranial nerve involvement resulting in deafness, blindness, hemi- or quadriplegia, muscular hypotonia, ataxia and permanent seizure disorders. Chloroquine and sulphadiazine are not known to cause deafness.

12.16. B C
Convergent squint is more common than divergent squint and is often associated with hypermetropia which can be corrected by the use of suitable spectacles. Untreated convergent squint can result in amblyopia. Treatment may have to be continued for a number of years and some children require surgery for a residual amount of crossing that cannot be controlled with glasses alone.

12.17. Which of the following statements about convergent squint is/are true?

A If surgery aligns the squinting eye, the vision in that eye usually improves spontaneously.

B Surgery should only be performed after patching treatment has improved vision.

C Retinoblastoma and congenital glaucoma often present with convergent squint.

D When it is alternating amblyopia is more likely to develop.

E Convergent squint has a better visual prognosis than divergent squint.

12.18. A child of 18 months presents with a nonparalytic convergent squint. Which of the following statements is/are true?

A The squinting eye moves to fix vision when the normal eye is covered.

B Hypermetropia is the most likely cause.

C Hypermetropia if present will improve with age.

D The squint will improve with age.

E The squinting eye should be occluded as part of the orthoptic treatment.

12.19. Which of the following statements about amblyopia is/are true?

A It is treatable until the age of 20 years.

B It is treatable until the age of 4 years.

C It is treated by occluding the good and the bad eye alternately.

D It is usually caused by squint or anisometropia.

E It is a cause of an afferent pupillary defect.

12.20. Which of the following is/are recognized causes of cataracts in childhood?

A Galactosaemia.

B Gaucher's disease.

C Congenital rubella.

D Down syndrome.

E Phenylketonuria.

12.17. B C
Most cases of convergent squint are due to disturbances of vision, such as hypermetropia, which require treatment with glasses or topical myotics. Aligning the squinting eye by surgery will not restore vision. The majority of patients respond to treatment with glasses, although some may require surgery for a residual squint. Retinoblastoma and congenital glaucoma cause visual disturbance which leads to convergent squint. A divergent squint has better prognosis than convergent squint. When due to esotropia it is alternating and vision is likely to develop equally in both eyes.

12.18. A C D
Convergent squint is usually due to refractive errors. When the normal eye is covered, the squinting eye moves in order to allow the patient to look at the object clearly. Other causes include visual defects such as cataracts and refractive errors. Although hypermetropia requires treatment with glasses, it improves with age. Only the normal eye is occluded for treatment.

12.19. B D
Susceptibility to amblyopia is greatest within the first 3 years of life and the risk lasts until full visual potential and stability have been achieved. Treatment after the age of 4 years is, therefore, unsatisfactory. Treatment consists of occluding the good eye. Anisometropia results in squint in order to suppress the image of the deviating eye and to avoid diplopia. If it is untreated it would result in amblyopia. There is no disturbance of pupillary reflex in amblyopia.

12.20. A C D
Galactosaemia is associated with raised levels of galacticol, which causes cataracts. In congenital rubella infection of the lens causes the development of cataracts. Children with Down syndrome are more likely to develop cataracts. There is no increased incidence of cataracts in children with Gaucher's disease or phenylketonuria.

12.21. Which of the following statements is/are true in relation to mental retardation?

A   Mental retardation occurs in more than 1% of the population.
B   The majority of mildly retarded individuals are at the upper end of socio-economic scale.
C   Dietary modification may prevent some forms of mental retardation.
D   Pregnant women with no immunity against rubella should be immunized as soon as they find out that they are pregnant.
E   Early treatment of congenital hypothyroidism may not prevent the associated mental retardation.

12.22. Which of the following statements is/are correct of neuromuscular diseases?

A   The Duchenne and Becker types of muscular dystrophy exhibit the same mode of inheritance.
B   Visible fasciculations are characteristic of the muscular dystrophies.
C   Distal distribution of weakness and sensory loss is characteristic of peripheral neuropathies.
D   Nerve conduction velocity is slowed in spinal muscular atrophy.
E   The serum creatine kinase level is always elevated in the early stages of Duchenne type muscular dystrophy.

12.23. A distended fontanelle is a characteristic feature in infants suffering from

A   communicating hydrocephalus.
B   meningitis.
C   non-communicating hydrocephalus.
D   vitamin A intoxication.
E   megalencephaly.

12.24. An 18-month-old baby presents with a 10-day history of refusal to walk and ill-defined pain in the legs. On examination he cries when his legs are moved and will not flex his lumbar spine. Tendon reflexes are brisk. ESR = 30 mm/l/h. Total white cell count $20 \times 10^9/l$ (65% neutrophils, 25% lymphocytes, 8% monocytes, 2% eosinophils). Which of the following diagnoses is/are likely?

A   Neuroblastoma.
B   Gullain–Barré syndrome.
C   Poliomyelitis.
D   Lumbar discitis.
E   Osteomyelitis of spine.

12.21. A C E
Mental retardation can be defined as a performance more than 2 standard deviations below the mean. It follows that 3% of the population will fall in this category. The majority of mildly retarded individuals are at the lower end of the socioeconomic scale. Mental retardation can be prevented by diet in many metabolic diseases: examples are phenylketonuria and galactosaemia. Rubella immunization should not be carried out in pregnant women as rubella embryopathy, although rare, has been observed following immunization during pregnancy. Although early treatment of congenital hypothyroidism will result in normal development in most patients, it does not prevent mental retardation in all cases.

12.22. A C E
The Duchenne and Becker types of muscular dystrophy are both sex-linked recessive. Fasciculations are characteristic of anterior horn cell disease. In peripheral neuropathies there is weakness and sensory loss distally. In spinal muscular atrophy, electromyography shows evidence of denervation of muscle including low potentials and fasciculations. Nerve conduction studies are within the normal range. In Duchenne muscular dystrophy the serum creatine kinase level is raised at birth and is 10 times the normal value at the age of 1 month.

12.23. A B C D
A distended fontanelle is seen in infants with communicating hydrocephalus, meningitis, non-communicating hydrocephalus and vitamin A intoxication (due to raised intracranial pressure). The fontanelle is normal in megalencephaly.

12.24. A D E
Pain in the legs and lumbar spine in neuroblastoma occurs due to bony metastasis. In Gullain–Barré syndrome and poliomyelitis there may be pain on pressure on the muscles but there is no pain in the spine. Deep tendon reflexes are diminished or absent. Lumbar discitis and osteomyelitis of the spine can result in local pain due to the inflammation and referred pain in the legs due to nerve root compression.

12.25. Abnormal EEGs are usually seen in

A   childhood absence epilepsy (petit mal).
B   infantile spasms.
C   in between breath holding attacks.
D   Rolandic epilepsy.
E   behaviour disorders.

12.26. Which of the following skin lesions is/are associated with central nervous system abnormalities?

A   Linear streaky vesicles in the newborn.
B   Vitiligo.
C   Adenoma sebaceum.
D   Café au lait spots.
E   Telangiectasia.

12.27. Which of the following statements is/are true of degenerative brain diseases?

A   The infant is usually normal at birth.
B   Most of them are autosomal recessive.
C   Tay Sachs disease carriers can be identified.
D   Subacute sclerosing panencephalitis is caused by the mumps virus.
E   Prenatal diagnosis of metachromatic leukodystrophy is possible.

12.28. Which of the following statements is/are true?

A   Ataxic cerebral palsy is accompanied by hypertonia in infants.
B   In cerebellar lesions the ataxia worsens when eyes are closed.
C   Spinocerebellar tracts are degenerated in Friedreich ataxia.
D   Ataxia is a recognized complication of phenytoin toxicity.
E   Ataxia is a prominent feature of post-varicella encephalitis.

12.29. Migraine consists of attacks of headache, characteristically associated with which of the following?

A   Visual field defect.
B   Neck rigidity.
C   Intolerance of noise.
D   Unilateral Horner's syndrome.
E   Vomiting.

12.25. A B D
EEG changes are characteristic in petit mal epilepsy (3/s spike and wave), infantile spasms (hypsarrhythmia) and Rolandic epilepsy (single spike or spike wave discharges in central or mid-temporal areas). EEG is normal in patients with breath holding attacks in between attacks (although there is slowing during the attack) and has no characteristic features in behaviour disorders.

12.26. A C D E
Linear streaky vesicles on the limbs which become verrucous and then depigmented are the first manifestation of incontinentia pigmenti in the newborn. Adenoma sebaceum, shagreen patches and hypo-pigmented macules are seen in tuberous sclerosis. Café au lait spots are characteristic of neurofibromatosis. Telangiectasia in the skin and conjuctiva are seen in ataxia telangiectasia. Vitiligo is a harmless sharply demarcated skin lesion which has hyperpigmented borders.

12.27. A B C E
Degenerative brain diseases are usually recessive. Most infants are normal at birth. There is progressive loss of previously acquired motor, sensory and intellectual functions. Measles virus has been grown from cerebral lesions of patients with subacute sclerosing panencephalitis which may appear many years after the initial infection. Heterozygotes for Tay Sachs disease can be identified by serum assay of hexosaminidase A. Prenatal diagnosis of metachromatic leukodystrophy is possible by measurement of arylsulphatase A in cultured amniotic cells.

12.28. C D E
In ataxic cerebral palsy, initially there is usually hypotonia and depressed tendon reflexes in infancy. Eye closure does not affect cerebellar ataxia. In Friedreich ataxia there is degeneration of spinocerebellar, posterior column and corticospinal tracts. Ataxia and diplopia are recognized complications of phenytoin toxicity. Cerebellar symptoms are common in post-infectious varicella encephalitis and have a much better prognosis if present without cerebral symptoms.

12.29. A C E
Classically, an attack of migraine is preceded by an aura which often consists of transient visual disturbances including field defects and zig-zag lines. Other symptoms include intolerance of noise, photophobia and vomiting. Neck rigidity and unilateral Horner's syndrome are not features of migraine.

12.30. Which of the following statements is/are true of cerebral oedema due to head injury?
A   Fluid intake should be restricted.
B   It is aggravated by retention of carbon dioxide.
C   It is aggravated by administration of corticosteroids.
D   It is associated with a rise in blood pressure.
E   It is associated with bradycardia.

12.31. Which of the following have more than a chance association with ventriculo-peritoneal (VP) shunts?
A   Moebius syndrome.
B   Subdural haematoma.
C   Pulmonary hypertension.
D   School failure.
E   *Staphyloccus albus* bacteraemia.

12.32. With regard to spina bifida (myelocoele)
A   prenatal diagnosis is possible.
B   the majority of cases develop hydrocephalus.
C   severe kyphosis and scoliosis are adverse prognostic features.
D   reflex activity is characteristically absent below the neurological level of the lesion.
E   the autonomic nervous system is not involved.

12.33. In a patient with hydrocephalus controlled by a shunt, which of the following may be produced by blockage of the shunt?
A   Papilloedema.
B   Headache.
C   Fits.
D   Irritability.
E   Failure to progress at school.

12.30. A B D E
Cerebral oedema due to head injury should be treated by restriction of fluids to two-thirds of maintenance requirements. Carbon dioxide retention causes vasodilatation and thereby aggravates the cerebral oedema. Corticosteroids may help to reduce cerebral oedema. Rise in blood pressure and bradycardia are recognized signs of raised intracranial pressure.

12.31. B D E
Subdural haematoma occurs in VP shunts if intracranial pressure is low. School failure may be the only symptom in children with raised intracranial pressure with a blocked VP shunt. Colonization of the shunt tubing and valve by *Staphyloccus albus* can cause recurrent bacteraemia. Pulmonary hypertension is a complication of ventriculo-atrial shunt, which is now rarely performed. Moebius syndrome (maldevelopment of cranial nerve nuclei and their nerves) is a developmental anomaly.

12.32. A B C
Prenatal diagnosis of spina bifida by ultrasound or by measuring alpha feto-protein is possible. The majority of cases develop hydrocephalus as a result of the Arnold–Chiari malformation. Abnormalities of the spine indicate that the lesion is high and therefore the prognosis is poor. Reflex activity is present below the neurological level of the lesion and the autonomic nervous system is involved.

12.33. A B C D E
A blocked shunt would lead to raised intracranial pressure and could present with papilloedema, headache, fits, irritability and failure to progress at school.

12.34. In the presence of raised intracranial pressure there may be
A   bradycardia.
B   bilateral sixth nerve palsy.
C   arterial hypertension.
D   somnolence.
E   no papilloedema in a newborn infant.

12.35. In a 2-month-old infant presenting with floppiness and developmental delay, which of the following would favour a diagnosis of spinal muscular atrophy?
A   Absent deep tendon reflexes.
B   A strong grasp reflex.
C   Decreased external ocular movements.
D   Predominantly diaphragmatic breathing.
E   Parents who are first cousins.

12.34. A B C D E

Bradycardia, somnolence and arterial hypertension are recognized signs of raised intracranial pressure. Sixth nerve palsy is due to the stretching of the nerve because of its long intracranial course. Patients with raised intracranial pressure may not have any headache. In the newborn infant there is no papilloedema because the sutures separate, thereby accommodating the raised intracranial pressure.

12.35. A D E

Werdnig–Hoffman disease is autosomal recessive and is characterized by atrophy of anterior horn cells. Onset may occur *in utero*. Early manifestations are poor suck, weak cry and weakness of face, limb and intercostal muscles. The diaphragm is spared. External ocular movements are normal. The grasp reflex is weak. The deep tendon reflexes are absent and the breathing is diaphragmatic. Later in the disease bulbar dysfunction, facial weakness and progressive respiratory failure ensue.

13 Psychiatry and social medicine

13.1. Common causes of school refusal in a 5 year old include
A   phobia about the school.
B   schizophrenia.
C   parental marital problems.
D   depression in the mother.
E   depression in the child.

13.2. School refusal in an adolescent is often a part of
A   separation anxiety.
B   schizophrenia.
C   anorexia nervosa.
D   severe depression.
E   delinquency.

13.3. Symptoms associated with anxiety in childhood include
A   excessive worrying and fears in normal social situations.
B   early morning wakening.
C   pseudo-maturity.
D   poor sense of self esteem.
E   attention-seeking behaviour.

13.4. Elective surgical operations should be avoided in children aged 1–3 years because
A   the infant is immunclogically vulnerable at that time.
B   the child may interpret the experience as an attack.
C   they may induce infantile autism.
D   the danger of separation trauma is highest at that time.
E   anaesthetic risks are higher.

13.1. C D

Causes of school refusal include parental marital problems and depression in the mother. Young children are rarely fearful of the school itself. Unlike adolescents, depression and schizophrenia in a 5-year-old child do not usually present as school refusal.

13.2. A B D

School refusal is a condition in which a fear of going to school is the superficial aspect of a fear of leaving the parent. In adolescents it is also associated with depression and may be a presenting symptom of schizophrenia. Delinquency can result in truancy but not school phobia. School refusal is not a feature of anorexia nervosa.

13.3. A C D E

A small amount of worry is normal in any new social situation but excessive worrying and fears are manifestations of anxiety. The child is often shy, timid and clinging, emotionally immature, over-dependent and has attention-seeking behaviour and poor self esteem. The child may appear to be more confident and competent than he or she really feels. Sleep problems are rare.

13.4. B D

Above the age of 1 year, the younger the child the more severe the distress of hospitalization is until the age of 3 years when it diminishes. Immunity is lowest at the age of 3–6 months. There is no relationship between infantile autism and hospitalization. Anaesthetic risks are no greater at this age than at other ages. A very young child will be unable to understand the logical reasons for the operation and may well experience and even remember the hospitalization as a major trauma.

13.5. Clinical depression in childhood
A   is often masked by psychosomatic or conduct symptoms.
B   is associated with withdrawal, isolation and loss of interest in usual activities.
C   is rarely associated with sleep disorder.
D   may lead to thoughts about death or suicide.
E   may be associated with hallucinations and delusions.

13.6. Which of the following statements is/are true of tricyclic antidepressants?
A   They are one of the major causes of fatal accidental poisoning in children.
B   They usually provide only temporary relief of nocturnal enuresis.
C   They are the treatment of choice for depression.
D   They are more cardiotoxic in children than in adults.
E   They exacerbate hyperkinetic syndrome.

13.7. Which of the following statements is/are true of breath holding attacks?
A   Consciousness is not lost.
B   Clonic twitching may occur.
C   Anticonvulsant treatment is indicated when frequency of attacks exceeds once a week.
D   Onset is rarely before the age of 12 months.
E   Ventricular asytole is an inconstant but recognized feature.

13.8. A 6-year-old who has temper tantrums
A   should be smacked.
B   should be allowed to have his/her way.
C   should have 'time out' for at least an hour.
D   should be ignored.
E   should have 'time out' for several minutes.

13.9. Truancy is often accompanied by
A   antisocial behaviour.
B   separation anxiety.
C   recurrent abdominal pain.
D   dysfunctional peer relationships.
E   panic attacks.

13.5. B D E

Depression results in a sense of lack of pleasure in life which results in withdrawal, isolation and loss of interest in usual activities, and persistent lowering of mood which leads to thoughts about death or suicide. In severe cases it is associated with hallucinations and delusions. Sleep disorders (insomnia or hypersomnia) are common. The concept of masked depression has lost currency, but co-morbidity is common in childhood psychiatric disorders.

13.6. A B

Tricyclic antidepressants cause cardiac arrhythmias, have no antidote and can result in fatal accidental poisoning in children. Their use in nocturnal enuresis results in temporary improvement, but the problem often recurs following cessation of treatment, and even during treatment. They are almost as effective as stimulants in hyperactivity. Cardiotoxicity is the same in adults and children. Tricyclic antidepressants have not been shown to be more effective than placebo in the treatment of depression in children and adolescents.

13.7. B E

In breath holding attacks, convulsions and loss of consciousness can result and signal the end of an attack. Ventricular asystole, although rare, may occur. Anticonvulsants do not prevent the attacks. Onset can be at any age.

13.8. D E

Tantrums are increased by attention. They are best managed by ignoring or by 'time out'. Punishment (smacking) or reward (allowing the child to have its own way) will perpetuate the problem. The period of 'time out' is not fixed but is dependent on the age of the child – a good general rule being one minute for each year of the child's age.

13.9. A D

Truancy is a form of antisocial behaviour in older children and adolescents. It is often accompanied by other antisocial activities such as theft, drug taking, sexual offences (including sexual abuse of younger children) and poor peer relationships outside of the delinquent gang. It is not a manifestation of emotional disorders, which include separation anxiety, recurrent abdominal pain and panic attacks. However, an emotional disorder may co-exist, as may hyperkinetic disorder and scholastic skills disorders.

13.10. Stealing by 5-year-old children
A   is sometimes learned from parents.
B   usually leads to delinquency.
C   commonly occurs at home.
D   is uncommon.
E   is a sign of parental neglect.

13.11. Behaviour therapy in children may utilize which of the following principles?
A   Reinforcement.
B   Transference.
C   Free association.
D   Time out.
E   Resistance.

13.12. The principle features of hyperkinetic disorder include
A   poor concentration.
B   hypersomnia.
C   obesity.
D   impulsiveness.
E   restlessness.

13.13. Good prognostic signs in a child with a conduct disorder include
A   poor self-esteem.
B   poor social skills
C   good scholastic aptitude.
D   success at sports.
E   development of a stable relationship or friendship.

13.14. A child with Asperger's syndrome will present with
A   failure to develop peer relationships despite ample opportunities.
B   inadequate use of appropriate non-verbal communications such as eye-to-eye gaze.
C   impaired speech development.
D   clumsiness.
E   good response to psychostimulant medication.

13.10. A C E

Stealing sometimes occurs in children of parents who boast of breaking the law (e.g. avoiding tax or exceeding speed limits). It commonly occurs at home, sometimes to invite punishment or attention as the child has a feeling of not being cared for. It occurs equally in all social groups. Almost all children steal something at some time.

13.11. A D

Principles of behaviour therapy include reinforcement (increasing a desired behaviour usually by some type of reward, emotional or material), extinction (to choose to diminish undesirable behaviour), 'time out' (temporary removal from a reinforcing setting) and ignoring (refusal to respond to undesired behaviour). Free association, transference and resistance are technical terms relating to psychodynamic forms of psychotherapy.

13.12. A D E

In children hyperkinetic disorder is manifested as restlessness, inability to concentrate (e.g. doing puzzles, construction toys) and impulsiveness. They may also be irritable and moody. Obesity and hypersomnia are not features of this syndrome.

13.13. C D E

Children whose conduct disturbance is limited to minor or isolated antisocial acts, whose relationships with other children are good, who are good at sports and show good scholastic aptitude have a better prognosis as each of these can be the basis of self-esteem and social skills development. Poor social skills and low self-esteem are indicators of poor prognosis.

13.14. A B D

Asperger's syndrome shares with childhood autism the features of impaired capacity to relate to other people through a sense of empathy and through non-verbal means and preoccupation with circumscribed subjects, rituals and stereotypies. Unlike autistic children, those with Asperger's syndrome have relatively preserved language skills but impaired motor development. Treatment should emphasize psychological support of the family and child, adaptation of the school environment and social skills training. Stimulant medication is rarely indicated and may even worsen behaviour.

13.15. Which of the following statements is/are true of childhood autism?

A   Onset occurs before the age of 3 years.
B   It is a disorder of communication.
C   Signs include lack of eye contact.
D   A well-developed delusional system is apparent.
E   There is avoidance of human relationships.

13.16. A 4-year-old non-speaking child is referred because of overall cognitive retardation. He makes no eye contact, does not respond to his name and panics at the sound of a lawn-mower outside. He is very active and walks on tip-toe, spinning a string between his fingers. Which of the following is/are likely to be true?

A   The patient will be disturbed if his familiar routines are interrupted.
B   The condition has been precipitated by acute intracranial infection.
C   Prognosis with psychotherapy is good.
D   The condition is more common in boys.
E   There is a strong familial tendency.

13.17. Which of the following is/are recognized features of anorexia nervosa in adolescent girls?

A   Amenorrhoea.
B   Hyperthyroidism.
C   High physical activity.
D   Fluid and electrolyte abnormalities.
E   Accurate description of body size.

13.18. Anorexia nervosa

A   only responds to family and individual psychotherapy.
B   is more common in girls than in boys.
C   is influenced by community values about diet and thinness.
D   is easily confused with endogenous depression.
E   occurs rarely in socially disadvantaged groups.

13.15. A B C E
Childhood autism usually presents before the age of 36 months. Such children have abnormal development of social relationships and language (leading to disorder of communication, lack of eye contact and avoidance of human relationships). Delusions are not a feature of this disorder.

13.16. A D
The stem suggests a diagnosis of infantile autism, which is more common in boys. Such patients often become distressed and agitated if their familiar routines are interrupted. It has no relationship with intracranial infection. Although the condition can be familial (2–3% of siblings are affected) the aetiology is heterogeneous. The prognosis with or without treatment is poor, although some specific behavioural disturbances can be addressed. The prognosis is better in children with higher intelligence and those with good speech development.

13.17. A C D
Clinical features of anorexia nervosa include excessive physical activity and dieting because of a morbid fear of being fat; accompanying this there is apparent misperception of bodily appearance (patient overestimating the size of thighs etc.) and amenorrhoea. Electrolyte imbalance results from vomiting, from water overloading and from abuse of diuretics or laxatives. T3 and T4 levels may be low with a normal TSH, in keeping with the patient's state of starvation.

13.18. B C
Anorexia nervosa is more than 10 times more common in girls than in boys and is more common in communities where there is great emphasis on body image. Treatment consists of individual and family psychotherapy, behaviour modification techniques and nutritional rehabilitation. Hospitalization may be indicated. Depression is not a primary feature of anorexia nervosa. The condition can affect all social groups, but is probably more common in the more affluent classes.

13.19. The differential diagnosis of a 14-year-old girl presenting with severe weight loss and amenorrhoea includes

A   depression.
B   anorexia nervosa.
C   anxiety.
D   bulimia.
E   subacute sclerosing panencephalitis (SSPE).

13.20. Child physical abuse and/or neglect should be suspected if

A   there is a delay in social and language skills with normal motor development.
B   there is growth failure without an organic cause.
C   a child is demanding and aggressive in the presence of his/her parents.
D   the parents' history of injury in a child is not compatible with findings on examination.
E   the child continues to fail to thrive in hospital.

13.21. The parents of a girl who has been sexually abused should be advised

A   that the child should talk about the incident until she has 'got it out of her system'.
B   that what happened was not her fault.
C   to make sure that further incidents do not occur.
D   that they will have to reassure their daughter of her worth and their love.
E   that the girl will have to give testimony in open court if the perpetrator is charged.

13.22. The persistence for years of incest between father and daughter is frequently due to which of the following?

A   Coercion by the mother.
B   The child's fear that she will not be believed.
C   The child's wish to protect her father from punishment.
D   The child's fear that revelation will lead to the break up of the family.
E   The child's trust in her father.

13.19. A B

In depression and anorexia nervosa there is severe weight loss and amenor-rhoea. Amenorrhoea is not a feature of anxiety and subacute sclerosing panen-cephalitis. Bulimia may be associated with great fluctuations in weight (of more than 10–20 kg).

13.20. A B D

Children who are neglected tend to have delay in language and social skills because of lack of stimulation. They gain weight inadequately but put on weight when they are admitted and observed in hospital. Normal children can be demanding and aggressive. Classically, the history given by the parents is incompatible with the injuries seen in an abused child.

13.21. B C D

In child sexual abuse it is important that the child be reassured that it was not her fault, and the parents still love her and hold her in high esteem. It is impor-tant to make sure that further incidents do not occur. If the child is asked to testify it is usually held in a closed court. Repeated talking about the incident will make the child feel guilty and embarrassed.

13.22. B C D

In the majority of cases, the mother is unaware of the incest. Children are extremely loyal to their family and are afraid that they may cause break up of the family if they mention it to other people. Children's early attempts to draw attention to the problem are often half-hearted, and because they are met with anger and denial they do not persist. Most children lose all trust in the parent that is abusing them.

13.23. Children who have been sexually abused frequently experience problems with

A ability to trust others.
B guilt.
C poor self esteem.
D frequent soiling.
E gender identity.

13.24. Enuresis in an 8-year-old boy who has been continent of urine between the ages of 4 and 5 years

A may be precipitated by a family crisis.
B does not require specific treatment.
C may have an organic cause.
D may lead to poor self-esteem.
E responds best to individual psychotherapy

13.25. Which of the following is/are correct?

A Nocturnal enuresis is more frequent in boys than girls.
B Diurnal enuresis is more frequent in boys than girls.
C Nocturnal enuresis is more frequent in first-born children.
D Nocturnal enuresis is a familial disorder.
E Primary enuresis may present at the age of approximately 4 years.

13.26. A 9-year-old boy presents with symptoms of nasal 'itching' accompanied by uncontrolled facial grimaces, and sniffling. This has occurred several times a day over the previous 4–9 months. Which of the following is/are likely?

A Attention-seeking behaviour.
B Attention deficit disorder.
C Obsessive compulsive disorder.
D Tic disorder.
E Psychomotor epilepsy.

13.23. A B C
Sexually abused children have difficulty in trusting others as they have lost trust in a close family member. They feel guilty as they feel they are perpetuating the relationship and have poor self-esteem because they feel valueless other than as a sex object. Soiling can occur but is not frequent. There is no problem with gender identity.

13.24. A C D
Enuresis in a child who has been continent before requires investigations. It can be precipitated by family crisis or may be the manifestation of some other disease such as urinary tract infection or diabetes mellitus. In the latter case polyuria results in nocturnal enuresis, although the child can be dry during the day. Psychotherapy will be of very little use in such cases. These children have poor self-esteem. Treatment will depend on the cause.

13.25. A C D
Epidemiological studies have shown nocturnal enuresis is more common in boys and in first-born children. It has a familial incidence. By definition primary enuresis is present from birth. Diurnal enuresis is more common in girls.

13.26. D
The description is most consistent with a motor tic disorder, comprising sudden recurrent, stereotyped movements accompanied in this case by some sensory symptoms. Transient tic disorders occur in about 10% of school-age children. Attention-seeking behaviour is an unhelpful term and implies deliberate misbehaviour. Tics are experienced as irresistible but can be voluntarily suppressed for periods of time. Tics are not an integral part of hyperkinetic disorder or obsessive compulsive disorder, but may co-exist. There is no evidence of obsessional thoughts or of anxiety on suppression of movements in this case, and the movements are typical of tics and not compulsive rituals. Consciousness is not impaired, excluding a diagnosis of psychomotor epilepsy.

13.27. Completed suicide in childhood and adolescence

A   is more common in girls.
B   rarely occurs before the age of 10 years.
C   is usually accidental rather than being planned.
D   may be associated with drug or alcohol abuse.
E   is more likely if there is a family history of suicide or depression.

13.28. Obsessive compulsive disorder in childhood

A   is fundamentally different to obsessive compulsive disorder in adulthood.
B   responds well to psychodynamic psychotherapy.
C   responds well to cognitive behaviour therapy.
D   interferes with the development of social relationships.
E   is more common in families where the parents are also obsessional.

13.29. The first child of a young woman has been born with signs of Down syndrome. When her medical attendant tells her and her husband the diagnosis, she rejects it angrily. Which of the following comments is/are appropriate?

A   This kind of reaction is abnormal.
B   This reaction is a manifestation of the defence mechanism of denial.
C   The mother should be left alone until she is able to accept the truth.
D   A series of interviews are necessary to help the mother to accept the diagnosis.
E   There is a genetic association between maternal psychopathology and Down syndrome.

13.30. A 6-year-old boy with normal hearing and no physical abnormalities speaks appropriately at home but says nothing at school either in the classroom or in the playground. Which of the following is/are correct?

A   It is likely that he has been disturbed by psychological trauma at school.
B   The condition is due to reactive depression
C   Speech therapy is of limited value in this condition.
D   The child's mutism is elective.
E   This speech disorder is indicative of early infantile autism.

13.27. B D E
Suicide in children under the age of 12 years is very rare. It is three times more common in adolescent boys than girls. Parents often suffer from psychiatric problems, especially depressive syndrome and personality disorders. It is usually planned and may be associated with drug or alcohol abuse.

13.28. C D E
Obsessive compulsive disorders in childhood are no different from those in adults. They respond best to serotonergic antidepressants and/or cognitive behaviour therapy and not to psychodynamic psychotherapy. There is a strong family history, two-thirds of parents showing obsessional tendency and about 5% obsessional disorders. Twin studies suggest a genetic influence in obsessive personality traits. Rituals may seriously interfere with socialization and development of peer and family relationships.

13.29. B D
The normal reaction to bad news is first one of denial followed by sadness, guilt and anger. The mother will need repeated interviews to help her to cope with the problem. There is no association between maternal psychopathology and Down syndrome.

13.30. C D
The stem suggests a diagnosis of elective mutism. The condition is not usually caused by problems at school, reactive depression or early infantile autism. It does not require speech therapy. These children are often somewhat anxious and have an overprotective family.

13.31. Adolescents with chronic physical illness

A   experience more psychotic episodes than healthy adolescents.

B   more often experience loss of personal control and independence than do healthy adolescents.

C   are less likely to comply with treatment than are chronically ill younger children.

D   cope better with their limitations if their family life is stable.

E   have poor self-esteem in more than 80% of cases.

13.32. A 5-year-old boy presents with night waking, accompanied by screaming, sitting up in bed, being inconsolable, but having no memory of the night's events. This behaviour has occurred once or twice a week for the last 6 weeks. The parents are very worried because he seems so distressed and the whole family's sleep is being disturbed. Which of the following would be effective?

A   Setting up a bedtime routine.

B   Extinction of sleep incompatible behaviours.

C   Prescribe diphenhydramine.

D   Reassurance, safety advice, and continue to assess the waking pattern.

E   Systematic desensitization.

13.33. A physically healthy 6-year-old boy presents with a history of inattention, behavioural disturbance, declining school performance and social isolation from peers. He has recurrent nightmares and has started wetting the bed. The symptoms commenced 6 months ago following the sudden death of his father. Your initial management strategy includes

A   tricyclic antidepressant medication.

B   behaviour therapy.

C   further family interviews.

D   psychostimulant medication.

E   individual interviews with the child.

13.34. Maternal postnatal depression

A   occurs in less than 5% of deliveries.

B   has been associated with cognitive deficits in young children.

C   may be detected by interviews alone.

D   is strongly associated with the lack of supportive relationship with the partner.

E   is strongly associated with economic disadvantage.

13.31. B C D E

Adolescents with chronic illness are more likely than children to be intolerant of the enforced dependency, particularly if their families do not appreciate how the illness interrupts their progress towards independence. Not complying with treatment is one way in which they may try to assert themselves as they feel loss of independence, which results in loss of self-esteem. There is no increase in psychotic episodes.

13.32. D

The case described is of night terrors, which occurs in 1–3% of children and generally resolves spontaneously by late adolescence. They are usually associated with CNS maturation rather than psychopathology. Behavioural management techniques are not useful in this disorder and pharmacological treatment is not recommended as a first line measure. Explanation, reassurance of the family and ensuring the physical safety of the child are of major importance

13.33. C E

The history is most suggestive of a reactive process centring around grief and emotional trauma. By addressing the underlying psychological issues with the child and family, facilitating the bereavement process and supporting a return to healthy family functioning, the associated symptoms of nocturnal enuresis, inattention, misbehaviour etc. should resolve spontaneously.

13.34. B C D

Postnatal depression affects 10–20% of women, with onset in the first 6 months following childbirth. The diagnosis is made on clinical grounds. The quality of important past and present relationships is associated with the level of risk for this disorder. Sequelae for the children include cognitive, language and behavioural difficulties, especially in boys. While financial stress may be a risk factor, postnatal depression occurs across the socio-economic spectrum.

13.35. Munchausen syndrome by proxy

A   is a rare infectious disease.
B   can manifest with a wide range of symptoms and signs.
C   is commonly associated with parental psychosis.
D   has a mortality rate of more than 2%.
E   is best dealt with by training the parents in basic nursing and medical procedures.

13.35. B D

Munchausen syndrome by proxy describes a situation where one person (usually a parent or other primary carer) induces or feigns in another (usually a child) signs and symptoms of physical illness and seeks medical treatment for this factitious condition. The complaints are widely varied and may change over time. The parent (usually the mother) is rarely psychotic, but has a very disturbed relationship with the child, poor self-worth and may have Munchausen syndrome herself. Further tuition in medical and nursing procedures may increase the risk of harm to the child. The mortality rate in published cases is around 10%, with a similar further rate of permanent morbidity.

14 Orthopaedics and musculoskeletal system

14.1. The upper age limit at which spontaneous resolution occurs is
A   2 years for bow legs.
B   4 years for outset hips.
C   5 years for internal tibial torsion.
D   9 years for knock knees.
E   more than 7 years for inset hips.

14.2. Which of the following statements is/are true in infants and children?
A   Newborn infants have flat feet.
B   Bow legs are normal in infants.
C   Knock knees are normal at 3–4 years of age.
D   Hallux valgus may be asymptomatic.
E   Curly toes are familial.

14.3. Bilateral knock knee (genu valgum) is
A   a normal limb posture from 2–6 years.
B   treated with shoe wedges.
C   painless.
D   best monitored by serial x-rays.
E   usually treated by splinting.

14.4. Talipes calcaneovalgus is of clinical significance because of its frequent association with
A   congenital heart disease.
B   syndactyly.
C   cleft palate.
D   congenital dislocation of the hip.
E   urogenital malformation.

14.1. A E
Infants are born with bow legs which straighten by the age of 2 years and develop into knock knees which resolve by the age of 6 years. Medial tibial torsion will not correct spontaneously after the age of 7 years. Inset hips continue to mould until the age of 16 years. Outset hips require orthopaedic treatment after the age of 3 years.

14.2. A B C D E
Newborn infants do not have well-developed foot arches and the feet appear flat. At birth the infant has bow legs. By the age of 12–24 months the legs have straightened and progress to knock knees. Adult configuration of legs is achieved by the age of 6–7 years. Hallux valgus is seen in adolescents, especially in girls, and is usually symptomless. The condition is progressive and may represent faulty development of the bones. Curly toes (some toes on top of others) are familial and are of no clinical significance.

14.3. A C
Infants have bow legs at birth which straighten by the age of 24 months and progress to knock knees. Persistence of knock knees beyond 6 years is abnormal and needs evaluation for an underlying abnormality. The condition is bilateral. It is painless and requires no X-rays.

14.4. D
Talipes calcaneovalgus usually occurs because of the position of the fetus *in utero*; this is also associated with congenital dislocation of the hip. There is no association of congenital heart disease, syndactyly, cleft palate or urogenital malformations with talipes calcaneovalgus.

14.5. Which of the following signs may be present in an infant with congenital dislocation of hips (CDH)?
A   Asymmetrical thigh folds.
B   Limitation of abduction of hips.
C   Absent femoral pulse.
D   Crying due to pain on movement of leg.
E   Delay in gross motor milestones.

14.6. Which of the following are associated with increase in risk of congenital dislocation of hip?
A   Family history of the lesion.
B   Breech delivery.
C   Talipes calcaneovalgus.
D   Carrying the baby on the back in a sling with hips abducted.
E   Myelomeningocoele.

14.7. Which of the following statements is/are true about slipped femoral epiphysis?
A   Peak incidence is between 5 and 10 years of age.
B   Bilateral slipping occurs in 15–30% of cases.
C   Operative fixation of the epiphysis is the treatment of choice in early epiphyseal displacement to prevent further slipping.
D   Two-thirds of patients are known to have had clicks on abduction of the hips in the neonatal period.
E   Avascular necrosis is a recognized complication.

14.8. Perthes' disease is
A   often manifest by knee pain.
B   most commonly seen after puberty.
C   a form of avascular necrosis.
D   indistinguishable from transient synovitis at the onset.
E   usually treated by surgery.

14.5. A B C
Clinically, the Ortolani or Barlow manoeuvre is used to diagnose CDH. Asymmetrical thigh folds should alert the examiner to the possibility of a dislocated hip, although they may be present normally. CDH is painless but causes limitation of abduction of the hips. Femoral pulses may be absent in anterior CDH. Gross motor milestones are normal.

14.6. A B C E
The aetiology of congenital dislocation of the hip is multifactorial. There are genetic factors and girls are more commonly affected than boys. It may be associated with other abnormalities such as talipes calcaneovalgus and myelomeningocoele. The association with breech birth is related to the position of the fetus *in utero*. The incidence has been shown to be less common in populations that carry their infants on the back in a sling with hips abducted, but is more common when carrying on a papoose board.

14.7. B C E
Slipped femoral epiphysis occurs in adolescent obese boys and is often bilateral. Avascular necrosis may occur as a result of disturbance of blood supply. There is no relationship to clicks on abduction of the hips in the neonatal period. Early fixation of the epiphysis will prevent further slipping.

14.8. A C D
Perthes' disease is avascular necrosis of the femoral head and occurs at the age of 5–10 years. It presents with limp and pain at the hip joint or referred pain at the knee joint and may initially be indistinguishable from transient synovitis because the symptoms and X-ray changes are similar. Treatment consists of allowing the child to weight-bear, but with the femur in an abducted position so that the head is well contained in the acetabulum. This is usually achieved with a long-leg cast in which the legs are held in abduction and medial rotation by a bar between the two casts (Petrie cast), although surgical procedures have been developed to keep the femoral head contained in relation to the acetabulum.

14.9. Which of the following may cause a limp and painful knee in a child?
A   Perthes disease.
B   Slipped femoral epiphysis.
C   Poliomyelitis.
D   Haemophilia.
E   Tuberculosis of hip joint.

14.10. Idiopathic scoliosis
A   does not usually progress after skeletal maturity.
B   is more common in girls than boys.
C   has a familial tendency.
D   bracing is best instituted at the time of skeletal maturity.
E   is usually accompanied by rotation around the vertebra.

14.11. Which of the following statements is/are true of torticollis due to sternomastoid contracture?
A   Restriction of rotation occurs towards the contracted side.
B   Jaw tilt occurs away from the contracted side.
C   Flattening of the face on the non-contracted side is observed.
D   It is not seen in babies delivered by Caesarean section.
E   Spinal abnormalities are found in more than 30% of cases.

14.12. Which of the following statements is/are true of a sternomastoid tumour in a 6-week-old infant?
A   It will resolve spontaneously (without treatment).
B   It will become malignant in approximately 2% of cases.
C   The patient will develop limitation of rotation of the neck to the side of the tumour.
D   The patient can develop neck tilt many years later in spite of initial complete recovery of neck movements.
E   Most patients need surgical treatment.

14.9. A B D E
Disease in the hip joint can cause referred pain at the knee. Therefore Perthes disease, slipped femoral epiphysis, tuberculosis of the hip joint and bleeding into the joint in haemophilia can all present with limp and pain in the knee. In poliomyelitis there is no involvement of the hip joint.

14.10. A B C E
The aetiology of idiopathic scoliosis is multifactorial. Some cases are autosomal dominant with incomplete penetrance. It is asymptomatic, familial and more common in girls. The progression of scoliosis stops or slows down at maturity and therefore bracing would be of very little use at this age. The lateral curve of the spine (which is due to wedging of vertebral bodies and discs) is accompanied by a rotation around the vertebrae and the ribs rotate posteriorly on the convexity.

14.11. A B
In congenital torticollis the head is tilted towards the side of the contracture and the chin is turned towards the opposite side. There is restriction of rotation of the neck towards the contracted side. Persistent torticollis may lead to asymmetrical development of the face and skull and results in poor development on the contracted side. Spinal abnormalities may cause torticollis but are not necessarily associated with congenital torticollis due to sternomastoid contracture. Torticollis has been observed in infants delivered by Caesarean section.

14.12. A C D
The exact aetiology of the sternomastoid tumour is not known, but it is thought to be due to an injury. The tumour resolves spontaneously and does not become malignant. Contracture of the muscle occurs and there is limitation of the rotation of the neck to the side of the tumour because of the unopposed action of the contracted muscle. The patient may make an apparent recovery but contracture of the sternomastoid may continue, which may result in development of a neck tilt subsequently. Most patients recover following neck physiotherapy and do not require surgical treatment.

14.13. Which of the following is/are recognized complications of cavernous haemangioma?
A   Cardiac failure.
B   Local gigantism.
C   Consumptive coagulopathy.
D   Malignant disease.
E   Bleeding.

14.14. A port-wine stain in an infant aged 1 month will
A   become worse over the next 1–2 years then regress.
B   indicate a risk of occurrence in 1 in 8 future siblings.
C   remain permanently.
D   probably become malignant if not excised during childhood.
E   respond well to treatment with carbon dioxide snow.

14.15. Which of the following statements is/are true of haemangiomas?
A   Strawberry naevi are not usually apparent at birth.
B   Strawberry naevi ultimately regress completely.
C   Facial port-wine naevus indicates a risk of seizures.
D   Thrombocytopenia is a recognized complication.
E   Corticosteroid treatment usually causes mixed cavernous capillary haemangiomas to regress.

14.16. Acute osteomyelitis
A   is most commonly situated in the metaphyses of long bones.
B   is unlikely in the presence of a normal X-ray appearance.
C   is most frequently caused by *Staphylococcus aureus*.
D   is often associated with a positive blood culture.
E   is best treated initially with benzyl penicillin while awaiting sensitivity tests.

14.17. The usual form of acute osteomyelitis of the tibia in a child
A   is associated with pain and pyrexia.
B   is located in the epiphysis.
C   is commonly associated with bacteraemia.
D   is commonly associated with mild trauma.
E   requires bone scan for early diagnosis.

14.13. A B C E
In cavernous haemangioma, cardiac failure occurs because of presence of arteriovenous fistulae, local gigantism is due to increased blood supply, and consumptive coagulopathy occurs because of thrombcytopenia and intravascular coagulation. Malignant disease is rare. Bleeding can occur but is rarely severe.

14.14. C
A port-wine stain is a mature capillary haemangioma and does not resolve spontaneously. There is no known inheritance and it does not become malignant. Scarring will result if it is treated with carbon dioxide snow.

14.15. A B C D E
Strawberry naevi may not be evident at birth. They tend to grow more rapidly than the infant and may attain large sizes before regressing completely. Facial port-wine naevi are sometimes associated with similar naevi in the meninges (and choroid), resulting in fits due to focal irritation. Cavernous haemangiomata trap platelets and cause thrombocytopenia. They regress when treated with corticosteroids.

14.16. A C D
Acute osteomyelitis is due to blood-borne infection and is situated at the metaphyses at the entrance of the nutrient artery. X-ray changes do not appear for a week after the onset of illness. The most common causative organism is *Staphylococcus aureus*, followed by *Streptococcus pyogenes*. Treatment should be commenced with penicillin and cloxacillin in combination because of the possibility of penicillin-resistant staphylococci.

14.17. A C D E
Acute osteomyelitis is a blood-borne infection in the bone which presents with fever and pain at the site of infection, usually located in the metaphysis at the entrance of the nutrient artery. Most patients give a history of mild trauma. Gallium bone scan will show increased uptake at the site of infection.

14.18. An 11-year-old boy has a 4-day history of increasing pain in the distal thigh with no history of injury. He is limping and the thigh is swollen, tender and warm. There is a small effusion in the knee joint, but gentle active movement of the knee is possible. Which of the following diagnoses is/are likely?

A   Osteomyelitis of the distal femoral metaphysis.
B   Septic arthritis of the knee.
C   Osteogenic sarcoma of the distal femoral metaphysis.
D   Juvenile rheumatoid arthritis.
E   Cellulitis.

14.19. Infants presenting with multiple fractures suggest the possibility of
A   active rickets.
B   achondroplasia.
C   osteogenesis imperfecta.
D   non-accidental injury.
E   scurvy.

14.20. Which of the following complications occur(s) more frequently in association with supracondylar fracture of the humerus than with other limb fractures?
A   Osteomyelitis.
B   Peripheral nerve injury.
C   Volkmann's ischaemic contracture.
D   Fat embolism.
E   Non-union.

14.21. Which of the following is true of infantile seborrhoeic dermatitis?
A   It is seen in the first weeks of life.
B   Scalp and flexures are involved.
C   It is often accompanied by *Candida* napkin rash.
D   The skin is usually dry and itchy.
E   It presents with blistering.

14.18. A C E

Patients with cellulitis over a joint or osteomyelitis have signs of inflammation and sympathetic joint effusion. Osteogenic sarcoma can mimic signs of infection. In septic arthritis and juvenile rheumatoid arthritis joint movement is absent or severely restricted.

14.19. C D

Although rickets may cause abnormality of the shape of the bones and greenstick fractures it does not cause complete fractures. In scurvy there is bleeding under the periosteum and dislocation of the costochondral junctions. In osteogenesis imperfecta there is bone fragility which leads to multiple fractures and deformity of the long bones. Non-accidental injury is characterized by multiple fractures at different stages of healing. In achondroplasia there is failure of growth of bone at the epiphyseal ends.

14.20. B C

Volkmann's ischaemic contracture is due to disturbance of blood supply to the forearm following supracondylar fractures. The ulnar nerve is involved because of its proximity to the site of the fracture. The other complications can occur equally commonly in any fracture.

14.21. A B C

Seborrhoeic dermatitis in infants usually occurs within the first month of life. The lesions appear in the flexural surfaces and over the scalp as cradle cap. It may be patchy or may spread to almost the entire body. There is usually superadded infection with *Candida albicans*. Lesions are usually non-pruritic. There is no blistering. The presence of weeping lesions with pruritus suggests the possibility of co-existent atopic dermatitis.

14.22. Which of the following conditions can be confused with nappy rash?
A   Moniliasis.
B   Psoriasis.
C   Urinary tract infection.
D   Infantile eczema.
E   Seborrhoeic dermatitis.

14.23. Erythema nodosum can be due to
A   streptococcal infection.
B   sarcoid.
C   drug hypersensitivity.
D   Crohn's disease (regional ileitis).
E   *Yersinia* infection.

14.24. Erythema multiforme is due to
A   drugs.
B   herpes simplex infection.
C   mycoplasma infection.
D   vaccines.
E   post-staphylococcal infection.

14.25. For the third consecutive year a 7-year-old boy develops an acute irritable hip syndrome during the autumn months. It settles completely after 5 days in slings and springs. Which of the following statement is/are correct?
A   The condition was probably preceded by an upper respiratory tract infection.
B   He is at significant risk of developing Perthes disease.
C   Slipped upper femoral epiphysis may occur during these episodes.
D   This condition is a common cause of refusal to walk in pre-school age children.
E   Aspirate from the joint will be sterile.

14.26. Which of the following is/are characteristic of juvenile rheumatoid arthritis?
A   Unexplained high fever.
B   Morning joint stiffness.
C   Skin rash.
D   Generalized lymphadenopathy.
E   Specific autoantibody.

14.22. A B D E

Moniliasis, psoriasis, infantile eczema and seborrhoeic dermatitis can all be confused with nappy rash. Closer observation of a lesion, e.g. satellite lesions in moniliasis, will establish the correct diagnosis. In urinary tract infection there is no nappy rash.

14.23. A B C D E

Erythema nodosum is due to localized hypersensitivity of the skin to bacterial protein (*Streptococcus*, tubercle bacillus, *Yersinia*) spirochaetes, drugs (iodides, sulphonamides, penicillin) and is also seen in chronic diseases such as sarcoid and Crohn's disease.

14.24. A B C D E

Erythema multiforme is characterized by erythematous macules, urticarial lesions, papules, vesicles and bullae. The most characteristic lesion is the target or iris lesion. It is a hypersensitive disorder as a result of immune complex formed in the body either due to drugs or microbial antigens such as herpes simplex virus, *Mycoplasma*, vaccines or *Staphylococcus*.

14.25. A D E

The stem suggests a diagnosis of transient synovitis, the aetiology of which is unknown. It has a strong association with viral upper respiratory tract infections. The patient may complain of pain at the knee. Pre-school children may refuse to walk because of the pain. It does not increase the risk of Perthes disease or slipped upper femoral epiphyses.

14.26. A B C D

Manifestations of juvenile rheumatoid arthritis include unexplained high fever (Still's disease), stiffness of the joints in the morning, skin rash, which may be evanescent, and generalized lymphadenopathy. Rheumatoid factor may be found but is not specific to rheumatoid arthritis.

14.27. Which of the following statements is/are true of Duchenne muscular dystrophy?

A   Antenatal diagnosis can be made.

B   Serum creatine kinase (CPK) is raised from birth.

C   Sitting up is delayed.

D   The knee jerk becomes depressed before the ankle jerk.

E   At least 10% of affected persons will have mental deficiency.

14.28. A boy aged 2 years presents with a history of delayed milestones, muscular hypotonia and depressed tendon reflexes. Which of the following statements is/are true?

A   A normal serum creatine kinase level (no technical error) excludes the possibility of Duchenne type muscular dystrophy.

B   Muscular hypotonia excludes the possibility of cerebral palsy.

C   Fasciculation of the tongue would suggest peripheral neuropathy.

D   Spinal muscular atrophy is a possible diagnosis.

E   Electromyography would be more useful in diagnosing a lower motor neurone cause than a cerebral cause for his problem.

14.29. Which of the following statements is/are true of Duchenne type muscular dystrophy (DMD)?

A   Fewer than 50% of affected people live more than 25 years.

B   Cardiomyopathy is a recognized feature.

C   There is an increased incidence of intellectual handicap.

D   The preferred treatment for scoliosis complicating DMD is a Milwaukee brace.

E   Investigations can confirm or refute the diagnosis at 1 month of age in babies at risk.

14.27. A B D E

In Duchenne muscular dystrophy serum CPK concentration is elevated at birth and during the preclinical phase. The onset is usually before the age of 4 years but may range from 1 to 10 years. There is no delay in sitting up and the proximal group of muscles are involved before the distal muscles (knee jerk becomes depressed before the ankle jerk). Mental deficiency is a recognized association. If the index case is known, antenatal diagnosis can be made in subsequent siblings by DNA analysis.

14.28. A D E

In Duchenne muscular dystrophy serum creatine kinase is raised at birth and markedly increased in the initial stages. It is low in established disease. In some forms of cerebral palsy hypotonia is the major feature of the disease. Fasciculation of the tongue suggests involvement of the anterior horn cells. EMG will show decreased potentials with lower motor neurone disease whereas no changes are seen in patients with cerebral problems. Spinal muscular atrophy is a possible diagnosis.

14.29. A B C E

More than 75% of patients with Duchenne muscular dystrophy die before the age of 20 years. The majority of patients have cardiomyopathy, which is the chief cause of death. The mean IQ of children with Duchenne muscular dystrophy is 80; 25% have frank mental deficiency. Serum creatine kinase values are increased even at birth in these patients. No treatment for scoliosis (orthopaedic or Milwaukee brace) is recommended as it will make the patient less ambulant and predisposed to pneumonia.

15 Drugs, accidents and poisoning

15.1. Which of the following statements is/are true of paracetamol?
A   It has no anti-inflammatory action.
B   It has been implicated in the aetiology of Reye's syndrome.
C   Toxic doses are known to cause hepatic failure.
D   It is the drug of choice for infants with fever.
E   It is contraindicated in patients with history of asthma.

15.2. Tricyclic antidepressants are useful in the treatment of
A   enuresis.
B   encopresis.
C   endogenous depression.
D   nightmares.
E   emotional deprivation.

15.3. Which of the following statements is/are true of sodium cromoglycate?
A   It is a bronchodilator.
B   It inhibits the release of mediators of the allergic reaction from the cells.
C   It is only useful in atopic individuals.
D   It is useful in children with exercise-induced asthma.
E   Therapy should be given during episodes of severe asthma.

15.4. Phenobarbitone
A   is known to cause agitation and hyperactivity in children.
B   has been shown to be effective prophylaxis in recurrent febrile convulsions.
C   is contraindicated for neonatal seizures.
D   has a half life of more than 12 h.
E   may interfere with a child's cognitive performance.

15.1. A C D
Paracetamol has analgesic and antipyretic activity but no anti-inflammatory action. It is excreted in the urine after conjugation to glucuronide or sulphate by liver. Toxic symptoms include vomiting, hypotension and sweating. Liver damage occurs after ingestion of large does (15 g). Reye's syndrome or analgesic nephropathy have not been recorded following treatment with paracetamol. It does not exacerbate symptoms of asthma.

15.2. A C
Indications for the use of tricyclic antidepressants are depression, nocturnal enuresis and chronic intractable pain. It has not been shown to be of any use in encopresis, nightmares or emotional deprivation. Contraindications are hypersensitivity and simultaneous administration of monoamine oxidase inhibitors. It should be used with caution in patients with epilepsy, cardiovascular disease, heart block, glaucoma, hyperthyroidism and urinary obstruction because of its anticholinergic effect.

15.3. B D
Sodium cromoglycate inhibits the release from sensitized cells mediators of the allergic reaction, viz. it inhibits the degranulation of mast cells which prevents both the immediate and the late asthmatic response to immunological and other stimuli. Given as regular prophylaxis it is useful in all forms of asthma, including that due to exercise. It is not a bronchodilator and is of no use during an acute severe asthmatic attack.

15.4. A B D E
Phenobarbitone is a long-acting barbiturate because of its slow metabolism, which results in a half-life of more than 12 h. Apart from sodium valproate, it is the only drug that is effective prophylaxis for recurrent febrile convulsions, although it has the disadvantage of causing hyperactivity in some children and may interfere with the child's cognitive performance. It is the first-line drug for treatment of neonatal seizures but it is not very effective in hypoxic ischaemic encephalopathy.

15.5. Which of the following statements is/are true?

A   The use of antibiotics in otitis media has reduced the incidence of intracranial infection.

B   Ampicillin may cause a fine macular rash which is of no clinical significance.

C   Tetracyclines are useful in young children.

D   Erythromycin may be helpful in *Mycoplasma* infections.

E   Penicillin is extracted from a rain forest plant.

15.6. Tetracycline is contraindicated in young children because it causes

A   bulging fontanelle.

B   gastrointestinal disturbance.

C   cholestatic jaundice.

D   inhibition of vitamin K synthesis.

E   dental discolouration.

15.7. Recognized side effects of phenytoin (Dilantin) administration include

A   ataxia.

B   hirsutism.

C   hypertrophy of the gums.

D   lymphadenopathy.

E   renal papillary necrosis.

15.8. Which of the following statements is/are true of methylxanthines (theophylline)?

A   The slow-release preparations are predictably absorbed from the gastrointestinal tract regardless of the presence of food.

B   Pharmacokinetics of the drugs vary considerably from patient to patient.

C   They cause stimulation of the central nervous system.

D   They stimulate intracellular adenyl cyclase production.

E   They are not universally well tolerated by children.

15.5. A B D
Antibiotic treatment of otitis media has reduced the incidence of mastoiditis and spread of infection to the brain. A fine macular rash which is not itchy sometimes occurs following administration of ampicillin. It resolves within a short time and does not indicate allergy. Tetracyclines cause discolouration of the teeth and are not recommended for use in children. Erythromycin has been demonstrated to be effective in treatment of *Mycoplasma* infections. Penicillin was originally derived from a mould, but most penicillins are now synthesized.

15.6. E
Tetracyclines are deposited in the teeth and bones. They cause discolouration of teeth in children. In young infants they can cause bulging fontanelle. Cholestatic jaundice is not a feature of tetracycline therapy.

15.7. A B C D
The side effects of phenytoin (Dilantin) include central nervous system manifestations (nystagmus, ataxia, mental confusion), gastrointestinal symptoms (nausea, vomiting and constipation), skin rashes varying from a mild rash to Stevens–Johnson's syndrome, bone marrow depression and lymphadenopathy, hirsutism and gingival hypertrophy.

15.8. B C E
The absorption of slow-release preparations of theophylline is altered when they are administered with a meal and may be accelerated or delayed, depending upon the product. The pharmokinetics of the drugs vary considerably from patient to patient and monitoring of blood levels is, therefore, important. Many children have severe gastrointestinal symptoms and central nervous system stimulation which prevents their administration. Intracellular adenyl cyclase production has not been demonstrated with the administration of theophylline.

15.9. Which of the following statements is/are true of penicillins?

A   They penetrate uninflamed meninges.

B   Phenoxymethyl penicillin (penicillin V) has the same spectrum of activity as benzylpenicillin.

C   They are recommended as prophylaxis for contacts of meningococcal meningitis.

D   There is no advantage of amoxycillin over ampicillin when given intravenously.

E   Ampicillin need not be discontinued if the patient develops a non-specific (macular) rash.

15.10. Which of the following statements is/are true of digoxin therapy?

A   It is the drug of choice for treatment of congestive cardiac failure in newborn infants.

B   Hypokalaemia potentiates its toxicity.

C   A high serum digoxin level indicates digoxin toxicity.

D   Anorexia (poor feeding) may be the only symptom of toxicity.

E   It takes at least 4 h for plasma and tissue equilibrium to occur.

15.11. In which of the following infections is erythromycin a suitable antibiotic?

A   Impetigo.

B   Urinary tract infection.

C   *Mycoplasma* pneumonia.

D   *Campylobacter* enteritis.

E   *Chlamydia* conjunctivitis.

15.12. Beta-blocking agents such as propranolol are contraindicated in the presence of

A   tetralogy of Fallot.

B   hypertrophic obstructive cardiomyopathy.

C   digoxin overdose.

D   asthma.

E   cyanotic congenital heart disease.

15.9. B D E
Although penicillins are found in therapeutic levels in the CSF in the treatment of acute meningitis, they penetrate the uninflamed meninges poorly. The therapeutic activity of phenoxymethyl penicillin and penicillin is the same, although differences in efficacy may occur because of the different blood levels that may be achieved. Many meningococci may be resistant to penicillin. Rifampicin is the drug of choice for prophylaxis in contacts of meningococcal meningitis. The spectrum of amoxyllin and ampicillin is the same: the advantage of amoxyllin over ampicillin when given orally is that the peak levels are much higher. The macular rash without itchiness that appears following administration of ampicillin is not allergic and does not require discontinuation of the drug.

15.10. B D E
The drug of choice for treatment of congestive cardiac failure in newborn infants is frusemide (and other diuretics). Hypokalaemia potentiates the toxicity of digoxin. Toxic effects of digoxin include cardiac arrhythmias and anorexia. Blood levels should be measured at least 4h after the last dose to ensure that tissue/plasma equilibrium has occurred. Drug levels are useful to determine whether adequate amounts of digoxin are being given rather than establish digoxin toxicity.

15.11. A C D E
Organisms that are sensitive to erythromycin include streptococci (which cause impetigo), pneumococci, staphylococci, gonococci, *Mycoplasma pneumoniae*, *Campylobacter* and *Chlamydia*. Urinary tract infections are usually caused by Gram-negative organisms which are not sensitive to erythromycin.

15.12. D
Propranolol is a beta-adrenoreceptor blocking agent which reduces the influence of excessive sympathetic nervous stimulation of the heart thereby reducing pulse rate, blood pressure, cardiac contraction and cardiac output. These effects are of therapeutic value in several cardiovascular diseases including tetralogy of Fallot, hypertrophic obstructive cardiomyopathy and cyanotic congenital heart disease. It is contraindicated in asthma, patients receiving hypoglycaemic agents or verapamil and in congestive heart failure.

15.13. Which of the following have been recognized as side effects of methylphenidate?

A Headache.
B Sleepiness.
C Anorexia.
D Habituation.
E Excess salivation.

15.14. In case of severe hypothermia

A rapid warming is potentially dangerous.
B the ECG may show a characteristic shortening of PR interval.
C warming is followed by a metabolic acidosis.
D plasma cortisol is reduced.
E hypoglycaemia may occur during rewarming.

15.15. Which of the following is/are associated with salicylate poisoning?

A Fever.
B Metabolic acidosis.
C Respiratory alkalosis.
D Pin point pupils.
E Hyperglycaemia.

15.16. Which of the following statements is/are true of childhood accidents?

A In developed countries they are the most common cause of death in children after the age of 1 year.
B The majority are preventable.
C They do not occur in children below the age of 6 months.
D Protection of the child is the ultimate solution in their prevention.
E Family social pathology would account for most accidents in children under 2 years of age.

Nervousness and insomnia are the most common side effects of methylphenidate. Others include anorexia, dizziness, headache, drowsiness and skin rashes. Habituation and drug abuse can occur. Excess salivation has not been reported.

15.14. A C E
Rapid warming following severe hypothermia will cause vasodilatation and circulatory failure. Hypoglycaemia results from the rapid use of the glucose and glycogen for the maintenance of body temperature. The metabolic acidosis is the result of the 'oxygen debt'. There are no characteristic ECG changes in severe hypothermia. The plasma cortisone levels are increased.

15.15. A B C E
Salicylates directly stimulate the respiratory centre, causing respiratory alkalosis. This is followed by dehydration, hypokalaemia and progressive accumulation of lactic acid and other metabolites resulting in a metabolic acidosis. Both hyperglycaemia and hypoglycaemia have been observed in severe cases. Fever has been observed.

15.16. A B E
Epidemiological studies have shown that accidents are the most common cause of death after the age of 1 year in developed countries, and the majority of them are preventable. Most accidents involving children under the age of 2 years are due to family discord, another sick child, house moving etc. Children under the age of 6 months may fall from 'change tables' or roll over in an unprotected cot. In the younger child protection, but in the older child education, is the solution in the prevention of accidents.

15.17. Which of the following statements is/are true of burns in children?

A   In developed countries burns are the leading cause of death in the home in children 1–4 years of age.

B   Loss of fluid, electrolytes and protein occurs into the interstitium of both injured and uninjured tissues.

C   Albumin should be administered as soon as possible.

D   Gastric ulcers are usually present in those patients who die.

E   Patients with low urine output need diuretic therapy.

15.18. Sudden unexpected infant deaths occur more commonly

A   in summer than in winter.

B   between 2 and 4 months of age than after 6 months.

C   in males than females.

D   sleeping in supine than prone position.

E   among infants that were of low birth weight.

15.19. Sudden infant death syndrome

A   can be diagnosed without a post-mortem.

B   affects all social groups equally.

C   after the age of 1 month it is the most common cause of infant mortality in developed countries.

D   is usually attributable to child abuse.

E   is often preceded by mild upper respiratory tract illness.

15.17. A B D

Accidents in the home (of which burns are most common) are the chief cause of death in children between the ages of 1 and 4 years. Fluid, electrolytes and protein move into the interstitium of injured and uninjured tissues ('third space') resulting in shock and electrolyte imbalance. Administration of colloids (including albumin) should be withheld for 12–36 h, when the capillary permeability of the injured area returns to normal. Gastrointestinal complications include stress ulcer and perforation; ulcers are almost universally present in those patients who die. Low urinary output is due to inadequate fluid therapy.

15.18. B C E

Epidemiological studies have shown that sudden infant deaths (SIDS) occur most commonly between the ages of 2 and 4 months during winter, in males, in prone position and low-birth-weight infants.

15.19. C E

The diagnosis of sudden infant death syndrome is one of exclusion and therefore cannot be established without a post-mortem. Epidemiological studies have shown that the incidence is higher in lower socio-economic groups. It is the most common cause of death between the age of 1 and 12 months in developed countries. Many infants have a history of a mild upper respiratory tract infection. By definition sudden infant death syndrome is not due to child abuse.

Printed in the United States
133561LV00003B/79/A